WHAT PEOPLE SAY ABOUT DR. BEALE . . .

"Dr. Beale is known as the foremost authority in the world on the treatment of obesity and overweight conditions in women of African descent. I personally know of his practice in Washington, D.C. and have consulted with him concerning the treatment of female patients of African descent in my own practice in Atlanta and Albany, Georgia. I am glad to see that he has put this information in book form so that the millions of overweight women of African descent who cannot come to our offices will have a guide to safe weight loss and better health."

DR. J. TOM COOPER
ATLANTA, GEORGIA

"We weight loss physicians who treat a large number of Black women in our practices have looked to Dr. Beale for guidance in this area for almost 30 years. His practice in Washington, D.C. is known as the largest weight reduction practice devoted primarily to Black women in the world. This book gives the reader the necessary information and resources to manage her own weight reduction program, preferably with the help of a caring, concerned physician or, if none is available, she can 'do it on her own.'"

DR. BILL NAGLER
DETROIT, MICHIGAN

"Three years ago I was diagnosed with multiple sclerosis and began taking medication. While the drug manufacturer and my neurologist stated the medication would not affect my weight, I steadily began to pick up extra pounds despite the fact that several times a week I was doing cardiovascular and weight training exercises. As my weight dramatically increased, I became really frustrated. I've always had intermittent weight issues, so for many years my diet consisted of fruits, vegetables, seafood, and chicken. I limited my sweets and carbohydrates, but no matter what changes I made to my diet and exercise program, I couldn't lose a pound. In fact, over a nine month period I trained for and ran two marathons. Guess what? The payoff for all my training was more pounds! I was at my wits end. Ultimately, I learned about Dr. Beale and began his program. From the very first week, I began to lose weight. Until Dr. Beale, I had no idea that some of the fruits and vegetables I had been eating were actually inhibiting my ability to lose weight. Thanks, Dr. Beale, for the education and for helping me to shed the unwanted pounds!"
MARIA
ROCKVILLE, MARYLAND

"Following the Dr. Beale diet, I lost eight pounds in less than three weeks, which was more weight than I have lost following any other diet or just reducing the amount that I ate. I just followed the yes and no list and actually felt like I ate quite a bit throughout the day. There was a food for all my cravings – especially my sweet tooth. The diet also caused me to eat healthier, which I have continued in the maintenance stage. I feel like I have much better control over my weight."
BLAYRE
SILVER SPRING, MARYLAND

"The issue of fad diets intrigued me enough to put three diets to the test as a television story. My station put three New Yorkers on three diets for one month. All of them lost weight but gained it back. I plan on passing Dr. Beale's fabulous diet along to one of the participants — a 33-year-old African American woman trying to lose weight after the birth of a baby. As the reporter for the story, I researched dozens of diets and I tried this one — believe me it works!!"

CATHY HOBBS
REPORTER/ANCHOR
NEW YORK, NEW YORK

The

Black
Diet Doctor's
Solution

For

Black Women

The

Black
Diet Doctor's
Solution

For

Black Women

Robert S. Beale, Jr., M.D.
Lisa M. Beale

Published by
The Diet Solutions, LLP
P.O. Box 65306
Washington, DC 20035-5306
Phone: 866-211-DIET
Fax: 202-478-0686
Website: www.TheDietSolutions.com

Authors' Pictures © The Picture People

Cover designed by Double Impact Designs

Printed and bound in Canada

10 9   8   7   6   5   4   3   2   1

ISBN: 0-9746307-9-9
Library of Congress Control Number: 2003098549

NOTE TO THE READER

This book is not intended to be a substitute for the medical recommendations of a physician, nor is it the intent of the authors to diagnose or prescribe. These pages merely reflect the authors' experiences, studies, research, and opinions; therefore, the advice and strategies contained herein may not be suitable for your situation. Consult with your physician before adopting any of the suggestions. Only he or she can determine whether or not this program is appropriate for you. Any questions, symptoms, or conditions requiring diagnosis or medical attention should be addressed by your physician. As in all health matters, his or her recommendations should be followed. While the publisher and authors have used their best efforts in preparing this book, they make no representations or warranties with respect to the accuracy or completeness of the contents and specifically disclaim any implied warranties of merchantability or fitness for a particular purpose. No warranty may be created or extended by sales representatives or sales materials. Neither the publisher nor the authors shall be liable or responsible for any health, welfare, or subsequent damage allegedly arising from the use of any information contained in this book.

DEDICATION

I dedicate this book to my grandfather, Robert Seate, a tobacco factory worker, who taught me to live my life with dignity, look everyone in the eye and not to be afraid; to my mother, Mabel Beale, a librarian, who taught me the value of education, to love books, to pray, and to trust in Jesus; to my little sister, Joy, who has kept me grounded in reality; to my teachers and advisors at Andover, especially Mr. Farrington, who taught me that all men are created equal and that I was to use my intellect for the good and betterment of all mankind, and that I could succeed at whatever I wanted as long as I worked hard and kept my eye on the goal; to my priest and spiritual advisor at Howard University, Father Ferrell, who gave me encouragement and wise advice throughout my college days; to my loving and lovely wife, Marilyn, who has been the source of inspiration and comfort for over 40 years of marriage; to my beautiful daughters, Lisa and Vicki, who have been a source of joy since the day they were born; to the bariatric physicians, Dr. Tom Cooper, Dr. Robert Johnson, and Dr. Fred Furr, who had the interest and took the time to help me begin my practice; to Mrs. Idelle Leavy, who has worked untiringly with me and our patients since we opened the practice in 1971; to my thousands of patients who have shared with me the pain, frustration, and depression that result from being overweight and the joy, happiness, and sense of accomplishment that result from losing and controlling their weight; and to my Lord and Savior, Jesus Christ, who has brought me all the way.

DR. BEALE

I dedicate this book to my father, Robert S. Beale, Jr., M.D., for his unconditional love and support throughout my life and my career. Daddy, I owe all of my success to you.

Love, Lisa

LISA BEALE

ACKNOWLEDGEMENTS

We would like to thank Idelle Leavy, Dr. Horace Laster, Dr. Robert Johnson, the late Dr. Peter Linder, Marilyn Beale, Vicki Beale, Joy Mitchell, Diane Danielson, Charisse Richardson, Deanna Turner, Cathy Hobbs, Marcia Parris, Mary Rogers, Blayre Josey, Sherry Deskins, Shaunia Carlyle, Aloysee Heredia, Sheila Mitchell, Dr. Yvonne Bronner, and Muv for all of their input and help.

ABOUT THE AUTHORS

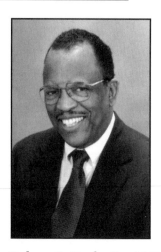

Robert S. Beale, Jr., M.D.

Robert S. Beale, Jr., M.D. was born in Prairie View, Texas, grew up in Durham, North Carolina, and was educated at Phillips Academy, Andover, Massachusetts, and Howard University, Washington, D.C. After serving in the United States Public Health Service, in February 1971 he opened an office for the private practice of family medicine in the Washington, D.C. suburb of Glenarden, Maryland.

He became interested in specializing in weight reduction in 1974 because he realized that many of the illnesses that he was treating such as diabetes, hypertension, heart disease, and arthritis were either caused by or worsened by being overweight. He joined the American Society of Bariatric Physicians (ASBP), an organization of physicians dedicated to the ethical treatment of obesity and eating disorders, in 1977.

Dr. Beale's practice in Washington, D.C. is the largest and most successful weight reduction practice in the world run exclusively by African-Americans. He has treated over 25,000 patients, the overwhelming majority of which are Black women.

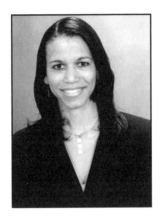

Lisa M. Beale

Lisa M. Beale, Dr. Beale's older daughter, grew up in Columbia, Maryland. She has a Bachelor of Science Degree in Computer Systems Engineering from Howard University and a Master of Science Degree in Computer Science from Johns Hopkins University. For many years, she had been an entrepreneur in the computer business until her father asked her to leave Los Angeles and return to Washington, D.C. to help with his weight reduction practice.

As Dr. Beale's daughter, she "grew up" with the practice and worked in the office in many capacities as a youth and young adult. She was glad to return to the practice and to the service of humanity, as she was not being fulfilled spiritually working primarily with machines.

She holds the titles of Director of Operations and Diet Counselor for Robert S. Beale, Jr., M.D. As an Affiliate Member of the American Society of Bariatric Physicians (ASBP), she has received and continues to receive organized training in weight reduction counseling.

Contents

Take Out and Fast Food
Drinking Water
When You Are Bored with the Food or Just Bored in General
When You Wake Up Hungry in the Middle of the Night
How to Deal with Cravings
Bad Breath
Constipation
Diarrhea and Gas
What to Do When You Have a Cold
Going on Vacation
Holidays, Birthdays, Anniversaries
Be Aware of the Feeder
Everyone Says I'm Beginning to Look Too Skinny
Walking – the Best Exercise
I Do Not Have Time to Exercise
Benefits of Working with a Bariatric Physician
Diet Pills from the Internet
Common Mistakes

PREFACE

This book was written to specifically address the unique challenges that women of African descent encounter when trying to lose and maintain their weight. Women of African descent may be natives of the United States, Canada, the Caribbean, Europe, Africa, Central America, and South America. It is proper and politically correct to use such terms as "African American," "Dominican," "Panamanian," "Jamaican," "French," "African," or "Brazilian." This book refers to women of African descent using the collective term "Black." It is by no means intended to minimize or disregard the race, ethnicity, and culture of the reader.

I have more experience in treating Black women for obesity than any other physician in the world. Until now, my methods and treatment philosophies have been available only to those in Washington, D.C. and nearby suburbs in Maryland and Virginia. With obesity among Black women at epidemic proportions, my daughter and I decided to write *The Black Diet Doctor's Solution for Black Women* in order to reach and help the millions of Black women around the world who suffer from obesity, who struggle to reach a healthy weight, and who, for reasons of geography, cannot come to my office.

This book is also a guide for the physician or other therapist who wishes to help Black women lose weight but may not be familiar with the facts presented here.

The weight loss programs are best followed under the care of a bariatric physician–this is a physician who is a member of the American Society of Bariatric Physicians and who has the interest and training to supervise a safe and maintainable weight loss program.

In my Washington, D.C. offices I have treated patients from Washington D.C., Maryland, Virginia, Pennsylvania, and West Virginia. Contact information:

Robert S. Beale, Jr., M.D.
1712 I Street, NW
Suite 604
Washington, DC 20006
Phone: 202-463-7872
Website: www.docbeale.com

I know of and have consulted with three other bariatric physicians in the United States who have the interest and experience in treating Black women for weight loss.

In the Atlanta and Albany, Georgia metropolitan areas contact:

J. Tom Cooper, M.D.
1234 Powers Ferry Road
Suite 104
Marietta, GA 30067
Phone (Atlanta): 770-952-7681
Phone (Albany): 229-439-0904

In the Detroit, Michigan metropolitan area contact:

Bill Nagler, M.D.
16311 Middlebelt Road
Livonia, MI 48154
Phone: 734-422-8040

In the New York, New York metropolitan area contact:

Gary Zisk, D.O.
8223 Bay Parkway
Brooklyn, NY 11214
Phone: 718-259-1979

If you are not in one of these metropolitan areas, these physicians cannot supervise you. To locate the bariatric physician nearest you, contact the American Society of Bariatric Physicians on the Web at www.asbp.org or by phone at 303-770-2526.

Being even a little overweight is dangerous to your health. Whether you have 10 pounds or 200 pounds to lose, you have the ability to lose weight by following the programs in this book. Even though it may be difficult at times, the results are important to your health and to your life.

DR. BEALE

Introduction

THE DIET SALON BY LISA BEALE

Our weight in many ways is similar to our hair. We were born with a certain type of hair and we were born with a certain type of weight. Some of us are lucky enough and have the genetics for easy-to-manage hair. For the rest of us, the elements of humidity, wind, mist, and rain have us searching for a permanent solution to the constantly changing and unpredictable weather.

We have many options from natural, to "permed", to braids, to a weave. Choosing a style and then getting our hair to that point does not always happen as fast as we would like. Braids, for example, may take up to ten hours. We would not even consider leaving the chair after two hours and then coming back a week later to finish. We sit there and knock it out.

We know that we can use expensive shampoo, we can deep condition, and we can keep the ends trimmed, but if we want our hair to be straight, we usually have to apply a permanent relaxer because our hair is not naturally straight. If we decide after years of straight hair to wear locks, then we have to be patient enough to let the "perm" grow out or be bold enough to cut it off.

Getting our hair done the first time is the hard part, maintaining is not as difficult. However, different styles require different types of maintenance. We would not go to a salon, get the perfect style, then for the next two months never look in the mirror or shampoo our hair. If we did, our stylist would look at us like we were crazy when we sit in her chair wondering why our hair is a mess.

No matter what style we choose and no matter how nice our hair looks, we know that it always wants to grow back to its natural state. We do not always have to go to the salon, but we at least have to look at it in the morning and we have to keep it clean. On those hectic days at a minimum, we simply pull it back into a ponytail, even if it is a clip-on ponytail.

We know exactly what products to use, what stylists to see, and how often to shampoo, condition, trim, and color in order to maintain our beautiful do's. We have silk pillowcases, silk caps, scarves, and a special way we prepare our hair before going to sleep so that it looks nice the next day.

It is a pain to deal with our hair and it can seem like a never-ending journey. As Black women, though, over the years we have learned to accept it and we have learned how to make our particular type of hair work for us.

We are constantly bombarded with television commercials and print advertisements featuring the likes of actresses and models of ethnic groups different from ours for the latest shampoo, conditioner, and hair styling gadgets. We know that most of those ads are not for us. We rarely even think about purchasing the products. Our hair is nothing like the women's hair in the ads. Manufacturers want us to believe that if we shampoo, condition, and blow-dry our hair every day using their products that it will be beautiful and free-flowing.

It seems to make perfect sense: We take a shower every day and so we should shampoo our hair every day. For millions of people shampooing their hair every day is essential. For most of us, though, if we shampoo and blow-dry our hair every day, it will dry out, it will be unhealthy, and it will not look good. Our hair is just different.

Collectively, we spend millions of dollars on our hair each year, but you essentially never see an advertisement for Black hair care products on mainstream television or in mainstream magazines.

We look to our stylists, our friends, and magazines targeted to Black women to learn about the latest styles, products, and techniques for our hair.

Given the fact that we would not even consider following the advice for non-Black-based hair care, why would we consider following the advice for non-Black-based weight loss?

Our bodies are different, just like our hair is different. It is okay to let our hair go every now and then because we do not have the time, desire, or energy to deal with it.

However, while a bad hair day will not kill you, obesity can.

We have read books, we have signed up for weight loss programs, we have joined gyms, we have trainers, we have cut down on fried food, we have oatmeal instead of a bacon, egg, and cheese biscuit for breakfast, we have popcorn or yogurt for a snack instead of a candy bar, and we have used skim milk, wheat bread, and low-fat cheese to make our favorite soul food dishes. However, the bottom line is that too many of us are still at an unhealthy weight.

Obesity among Black women has reached epidemic proportions.

All you have to do is sit in church, the salon, a concert, or around family members to see that this is true.

With so much information about the dangers of obesity and so many "solutions" on the market, why are so many of us still obese? The answer is that, through no fault of our own, we have been listening to the wrong people. We had to work with what we have been given. We were left to take the advice of non-authorities. The popular and nationally advertised weight loss products, plans, diets, exercise regimens, and books are not specifically designed for Black women by Black weight loss physicians who understand the physiology, psychology, and sociology of Black women.

Dr. Beale is the authority.

Dr. Beale has been treating obese and overweight patients since 1974. His practice in Washington, D.C. is the largest and most successful weight reduction practice in the world run exclusively by African Americans. He has treated over 25,000 patients, the overwhelming majority of which are Black women.

This book clears up all the myths and mistakes Black women make when trying to lose weight. The information comes primarily from the authors' own personal experiences with these patients and offers the first definitive how-to guide for Black women who want to lose weight permanently and be healthier.

While you are reading this book and implementing the program to lose and permanently maintain a healthy weight, keep in mind that your weight is like your hair.

◆ Based on genetics, you were born with a certain type of hair and you were born with a certain type of weight. Your hair type is not your fault and your weight is not your fault.

◆ Some people have naturally straight hair and some people are naturally thin. On the other hand, some people have naturally curly hair and some people naturally weigh 220 pounds. Curly hair will not harm you, but a weight of 220 pounds will.

◆ For some, having and maintaining a nice hairstyle is not a challenge while for others it is a constant struggle. For some, being at a healthy weight is not a challenge while for others it is a constant struggle.

◆ Your hair changes as you get older, it may become gray and it may become thin. Your weight changes as you get older. Child birth, age, illness, and menopause can be triggers for weight gain.

◆ It takes time and patience to get your hair to the desired style. It takes time and patience to get to a healthy weight.

◆ Once your hair is in the desired style, you have to maintain it because it always wants to grow back to its natural state. Maintaining is not nearly as challenging, but you have to do some things to keep your hair healthy. Once a healthy weight is reached, you have to follow the program in this book to maintain it. Your weight always wants to grow back to its natural state. You will not have to "diet" everyday, but you will have to follow the Maintenance Program to stay at a healthy weight.

◆ Different hairstyles require different types of maintenance. Once you reach a healthy weight, it becomes a personal decision as to how small you want to get. It takes more effort to maintain a weight of 140 pounds than it does to maintain a weight of 150 pounds.

◆ You can keep your hair clean, trimmed, and deep conditioned, but in most cases, if you want your hair straight, you must use a permanent relaxer. You can cut out fried food, eat healthy, and get plenty of exercise, but if you want to permanently lose weight, you have to follow the program outlined in this book. It is a two-step process. The first step is "Eating to Lose" and the second is "Eating to Maintain."

◆ Taking the advice of a stylist who does not understand the care and maintenance of Black women's hair will not likely get your hair to a healthy and manageable condition. Taking the advice of a non-expert, especially a non-physician, who does not understand the physiology, psychology and sociology of Black women will not likely get your weight to a healthy and manageable condition.

In addition, while heavy resistance exercise with weights, riding the bicycle, running, stair climbing, high impact aerobics, and squats may help non-Black women and men lose weight, sometimes the opposite happens for us. Think about the slaves who used to work in the fields. Now that was some exercise–lifting, bending, sweating, and the burning of many calories. Those were usually not small women.

Most Black women do not have the genetic makeup that allows them to engage in heavy exercise and lose all of their excess weight at the same time. You will be very strong and solid with that kind of exercise regimen, but you will probably not reach your desired, healthy weight.

Most importantly, remember that you are not a dieting machine.

Life does not stop because you are trying to lose weight. Throughout this book, we will also provide you with strategies to deal with everyday life. You are on a journey and there will be challenges along the way. Do not beat yourself up if you are not perfect with the diet every day or even every week. You will get back on track and you will get through it.

Dr. Beale is a Black physician who has treated thousands of Black women for obesity. He is your expert coach. You, however, will deserve full credit for your dedication and hard work in reaching your goal.

> *The race is not given to the swift nor the battle given to the strong, but to she who endures to the end.*

HELLO, STRANGER

To myself

Hey, you, there in the mirror staring back at me, I see the
hard stares, glaring clearly, deservedly back at me, I look at
you every day and pray for another.
Another face to have look back at me.
For I can't see that beautiful stranger staring back at me.
I can't tell why beauty lies, "Oh, it's not your hips; it's not
your thighs. It's only your mind that truly matters."
But to me it seems it's all just chit chatter.
Hello, stranger, I see you, putting yourself down again be-
cause some fool out on the street laughed at the size of
your backside again.
There's no one out here perfect in the world.
So we put each other down to make ourselves pearls.
Hey, stranger, don't worry about the perfect world, huh it
will never be.
I think that stranger in the mirror...That stranger is me.

Tamika Nikesha Armstrong

Ms. Tamika Armstrong is a patient of Dr. Beale, and an aspiring
poet and novelist. She wrote *Hello, Stranger* to express the feelings, trials, and discovery of self of an overweight woman in today's
society. She says, "To lose weight has been an uphill battle, but
anything worth having is worth fighting for."

Hello, Stranger conveys the sense of helplessness and despair that many Black women feel as they try to lose weight. No more do you need to feel this way. There is hope. The methods outlined in this book have worked on thousands of others, and they can work for you.

One

BLACK WOMEN AND WEIGHT

Your Weight Is Not Your Fault

Y our height is not your fault, your eye color is not your fault, the shape of your nose is not your fault, the texture of your hair is not your fault, your weight is not your fault.

Because of your genetic makeup your height naturally occurred, your eye color naturally occurred, the shape of your nose naturally occurred, the texture of your hair naturally occurred, your weight naturally occurred. You did not do anything right or wrong to get the body you have.

But you can change nature. You can wear heels to make you taller, you can wear contacts to make your eyes light brown, you can have plastic surgery to make your nose thinner, and you can put a relaxer in your hair to make it straight.

These are all solutions to change the body that nature gave you. Some of these solutions are more invasive or longer lasting than others, but the decision to make these changes is up to you.

You can permanently change the weight that is naturally occurring in you by following the *Weight Loss Programs* in Chapter 3 and the *Maintenance Program* in Chapter 5.

Hereditary Obesity Based on the Study of Rats

Most of the research that supports the connection between heredity and weight comes from rat studies. In the 1950s and 1960s, researchers were trying to make obese rats for their studies by feeding normal rats large quantities of fattening foods. They found that most rats did not gain sufficient weight to be considered obese and were hence deemed unsuitable for these studies. Those that did gain weight lost it rapidly when high calorie feed was replaced with normal feed.

However, some rats did gain weight and kept it on when fed an essentially normal diet. Researchers mated these rats and got mostly obese offspring. Then they discovered genetic components in these rats that seemed to be responsible for obesity.

Two prevalent strains of genetically obese rats were developed by breeding rats that were spontaneously obese with other rats that were spontaneously obese. The two strains are the Zucker rat, developed by Drs. Theodore and Lois Zucker at the Laboratory of Comparative Pathology at Stow, Massachusetts in the 1960s, and the Koletsky strain developed by Dr. Simon Koletsky at Case Western Reserve University School of Medicine in 1969. These genetically obese rats are now available for sale to scientists who want to study obesity and its treatment.

Please remember that data derived from rats are not always applicable to humans. Humans and rats are not always the same, but rats are easier to study than humans because rats can be bred at will, can be observed constantly, and can be given potentially dangerous drugs. Rats can also be sacrificed and autopsied without concern. Researchers cannot do those things with humans. The rat studies proved that there is a genetic basis for obesity and, in some cases, researchers feel that they have identified a single gene causing obesity in some rats.

The Single-Gene Theory

The single-gene theory for obesity in humans has not been proven, but research is ongoing. In fact, researchers are discovering that there may be over 250 genetic markers for obesity. The practical application for studying the genetic basis for obesity is in providing an explanation to those who have tried to lose weight and have not been successful. The studies also provide information for selecting feeding plans for children and infants, depending on whether or not they carry the gene(s) for obesity.

Permanent Weight Loss, a Two-Step Process

First you must "Eat to Lose" to get to your goal weight, and second you must "Eat to Maintain" in order to stay at your goal weight.

Step 1 "Eat To Lose" – When we speak of losing weight, we actually mean that we want to lose fat. We do not want our liver to get smaller, or our bones to get thinner, or our brain to shrink. We just want to lose fat. It is the goal of our weight loss programs to lose as much fat as possible and spare as much lean tissue as possible.

The only way to lose fat is to force the body to use it as fuel or a source of energy for the body. Energy is used here as a synonym for "source of fuel". The body will not use its own tissue (fat is a living tissue) as a source of fuel unless it has no other choice. The body will use lettuce as fuel before it uses stored fat.

Therefore, a weight reduction program must force the body to use its own tissue if the program is to work. In other words, you must give your body less food than it needs. The result is that now your body will be forced to find its source of energy elsewhere. An example of "elsewhere" is the fat on your thighs. This is how you lose weight.

Living on one's own tissue is not normal. Hence, losing weight is not a normal act. In other words, in order to lose weight, you must force your body to commit an unnatural or abnormal act. You are forcing yourself into an abnormal physiological state. It is normal to live on food, store some as fat, and eliminate the rest as waste. It is not normal to live partly on food and partly on your own tissue (fat). Our programs teach you how to remain healthy while living temporarily in an abnormal physiological state.

Chapter 3 *Weight Loss Programs* outlines how to "eat to lose." Chapter 4 *Weight Loss Strategies* provides suggestions for dealing with everyday life while you are on the *Weight Loss Program*.

The positive side of this is that you will not have to "eat to lose" forever. Once you reach your goal, you move on to Step 2.

Step 2 "Eat To Maintain" - Maintaining your weight is not an unnatural act. You are not living on your own tissue (fat), instead you are living on food, however you have to have the correct strategy to avoid the manufacture of new fat. This is simply a strategic issue, not an unnatural physiology issue. It is much easier to maintain a weight loss than it is to lose weight.

You must follow the *Maintenance Program* outlined in Chapter 5 in order to stay at your goal weight. You will not have to "diet" every day. You will be able to enjoy your favorite foods, just not at every meal. As with many things in life, it is all about moderation.

You already maintain your body in many ways. You take a shower and brush your teeth no matter how clean you were yesterday; you shampoo, condition, trim, and get occasional touch ups no matter how nice your hair looked when you left the salon; you shave your legs no matter how smooth they were three days ago; and you get a fill for your nails no matter how perfectly sculpted they were when you had them applied.

None of these are too difficult, but you must do them. You know it is just a part of your life and part of your routine because your body always wants to grow back to its "natural" state.

Implementing your weight *Maintenance Program* will not be too difficult, but you must do it. It will become a part of your life and a part of your routine because your body always wants to grow back to its "natural" state.

Healthy Weight Versus Goal Weight

Body Mass Index (BMI)
A "Healthy Weight" is a range based on a height-weight system called Body Mass Index (BMI). BMI is a measure which takes into account your height and weight to gauge total body fat.

The BMI metric formula is your weight in kilograms divided by your height in meters squared.

$$BMI = Weight \text{ [in kilograms]} / (Height \text{ [in meters]})^2$$

The BMI pounds and inches formula is your weight in pounds times 704.5 divided by your height in inches squared.

$$BMI = (Weight \text{ [in pounds]} * 704.5) / (Height \text{ [in inches]})^2$$

Defining Obesity

"Obesity" is defined as an excessively high amount of body fat relative to lean body mass. "Overweight" is defined as a high body weight relative to height. The National Institutes of Health uses the following BMI guidelines:

◆ **Healthy Weight** - BMI between 19 and 24.9.

◆ **Overweight** - BMI between 25 and 29.9.

◆ **Obese** - BMI of 30 or higher.

◆ **Seriously Obese** – BMI of 40 or higher.

Defining Your Milestones

You will have several milestones along the way. Reaching a milestone is an incredible accomplishment that will make you very proud. You will feel better, sleep better, breathe better, get around better, and generally be healthier for every 10 pounds you lose.

Your Goal Weight may be defined anywhere in the weight ranges for Milestone #1, Milestone #2, or Milestone #3.

BMI Chart–Healthy Weight

Healthy Weight						
BMI	19	20	21	22	23	24
Height (ft.,in.)	Body Weight (pounds)					
4' 10"	91	96	100	105	110	115
4' 11"	94	99	104	109	114	119
5' 0"	97	102	107	112	118	123
5' 1"	100	106	111	116	122	127
5' 2"	104	109	115	120	126	131
5' 3"	107	113	118	124	130	135
5' 4"	110	116	122	128	134	140
5' 5"	114	120	126	132	138	144
5' 6"	118	124	130	136	142	148
5' 7"	121	127	134	140	146	153
5' 8"	125	131	138	144	151	158
5' 9"	128	135	142	149	155	162
5' 10"	132	139	146	153	160	167
5' 11"	136	143	150	157	165	172
6' 0"	140	147	154	162	169	177
6' 1"	144	151	159	166	174	182
6' 2"	148	155	163	171	179	186
6' 3"	152	160	168	176	184	192

BMI Chart–Overweight
Moderate Health Risks

Overweight					
BMI	25	26	27	28	29
Height (ft.,in.)	Body Weight (pounds)				
4' 10"	119	124	129	134	138
4' 11"	124	128	133	138	143
5' 0"	128	133	138	143	148
5' 1"	128	137	143	148	153
5' 2"	136	142	147	153	158
5' 3"	141	146	152	158	163
5' 4"	145	151	157	163	169
5' 5"	150	156	162	168	174
5' 6"	155	161	167	173	179
5' 7"	159	166	172	178	185
5' 8"	164	171	177	184	190
5' 9"	169	176	182	189	196
5' 10"	174	181	188	195	202
5' 11"	179	186	193	200	208
6' 0"	184	191	199	206	213
6' 1"	189	197	204	212	219
6' 2"	194	202	210	218	225
6' 3"	200	208	216	224	232

BMI Chart–Seriously Overweight
Increased Risk of Health Problems

Obese									
BMI	30	31	32	33	34	35	36	37	38	39
Height (ft.,in.)	Body Weight (pounds)								
4' 10"	143	148	153	158	162	167	172	177	181	186
4' 11"	148	153	158	163	168	173	178	183	188	193
5' 0"	153	158	163	168	174	179	184	189	194	199
5' 1"	158	164	169	174	180	185	190	195	201	206
5' 2"	164	169	175	180	186	191	196	202	207	213
5' 3"	169	175	180	186	191	197	203	208	214	220
5' 4"	174	180	186	192	197	204	209	215	221	227
5' 5"	180	186	192	198	204	210	216	222	228	234
5' 6"	186	192	198	204	210	216	223	229	235	241
5' 7"	191	198	204	211	217	223	230	236	242	249
5' 8"	197	203	210	216	223	230	236	243	249	256
5' 9"	203	209	216	223	230	236	243	250	257	263
5' 10"	209	216	222	229	236	243	250	257	264	271
5' 11"	215	222	229	236	243	250	257	265	272	279
6' 0"	221	228	235	242	250	257	265	272	279	287
6' 1"	227	235	242	250	257	265	272	280	288	295
6' 2"	233	241	249	256	264	272	280	287	295	303
6' 3"	240	248	256	264	272	279	287	295	303	311

BMI Chart–Seriously Obese
Very High Risk of Health Problems

Seriously Obese									
BMI	40	41	42	43	44	45	46	47	48	49
Height (ft.,in.)	Body Weight (pounds)									
4' 10"	191	196	201	205	210	215	220	224	229	234
4' 11"	198	203	208	212	217	222	227	232	237	242
5' 0"	204	209	215	220	225	230	235	240	245	250
5' 1"	211	217	222	227	232	238	243	248	254	259
5' 2"	218	224	229	235	240	246	251	256	262	267
5' 3"	225	231	237	242	248	254	259	265	270	278
5' 4"	232	238	244	250	256	262	267	273	279	285
5' 5"	240	246	252	258	264	270	276	282	288	294
5' 6"	247	253	260	266	272	278	284	291	297	303
5' 7"	255	261	268	274	280	287	293	299	306	312
5' 8"	262	269	276	282	289	295	302	308	315	322
5' 9"	270	277	284	291	297	304	311	318	324	331
5' 10"	278	285	292	299	306	313	320	327	334	341
5' 11"	286	293	301	308	315	322	329	338	343	351
6' 0"	294	302	309	316	324	331	338	346	353	361
6' 1"	302	310	318	325	333	340	348	355	363	371
6' 2"	311	319	326	334	342	350	358	365	373	381
6' 3"	319	327	335	343	351	359	367	375	383	391

Your Goal Weight is your own personal decision as long as it falls within the weight ranges of the Milestones. There is absolutely nothing wrong with having curves and a little meat on your bones, but there is also nothing wrong with wanting to be thin.

Milestone #1 - At an absolute minimum, you should follow the *Weight Loss Programs* in Chapter 3 until you are out of the "Seriously Obese" and "Obese" BMI ranges. The risk of death from many causes is increased from 50% to 150% when you are obese.

Milestone #2 – Get as close to the "Healthy Weight" BMI range as possible. You are still at a moderate health risk for many diseases in the "Overweight" BMI range. In addition, as you get older, it becomes more difficult for your body's frame to carry those extra pounds.

Milestone #3 – You may not have a Milestone #3, but you may decide that you want to have a BMI of 21 so you can fit into smaller size clothes.

You Must Reach Milestone #1.

Obesity is killing Black women.

It is a harsh statement, but unfortunately obesity among Black women has reached epidemic proportions. The primary concern of obesity is one of health and not one of appearance.

According to the Surgeon General's *Call To Action* here are the health consequences associated with obesity:

◆ Premature Death
  - An estimated 300,000 deaths per year may be attributable to obesity.

  - The risk of death rises with increasing weight.

- Individuals who are obese have a 50% to 100% increased risk of premature death from all causes, compared to individuals with a healthy weight.

◆ Heart Disease
  - The incidence of heart disease (heart attack, congestive heart failure, sudden cardiac death, angina or chest pain, and abnormal heart rhythm) and strokes are increased in persons who are overweight or obese.

  - High blood pressure is twice as common in adults who are obese than in those who are at a healthy weight.

  - Obesity is associated with elevated triglycerides (blood fat) and decreased HDL cholesterol (good cholesterol).

◆ Diabetes
  - A weight gain of 11 to 18 pounds increases a person's risk of developing type 2 diabetes to twice that of individuals who have not gained weight.

  - Over 80% of people with diabetes are overweight or obese.

◆ Cancer
  - Overweight and obesity are associated with an increased risk for some types of cancer including endometrial (cancer of the lining of the uterus), colorectal, gall bladder, kidney, and postmenopausal breast cancer.

  - Women gaining more than 20 pounds from age 18 to midlife double their risk of postmenopausal breast cancer, compared to women whose weight remains stable.

◆ Breathing Problems
  - Sleep apnea (interrupted breathing while sleeping) is more common in obese persons.

  - Obesity is associated with a higher prevalence of asthma.

◆ Arthritis
  - For every two-pound increase in weight, the risk of developing arthritis is increased by 9% to 13%.

  - Symptoms of arthritis can improve with weight loss.

◆ Reproductive Complications
  - Complications of pregnancy
    * Obesity during pregnancy is associated with an increased risk of death in both the baby and the mother. Obesity also increases the risk of maternal high blood pressure by 10 times.

    * In addition to many other complications, women who are obese during pregnancy are more likely to have gestational diabetes and problems with labor and delivery.

    * Infants born to women who are obese during pregnancy are more likely to be high birth weight and, therefore, may face a higher rate of Cesarean section delivery and low blood sugar (which can be associated with brain damage and seizures).

    * Obesity during pregnancy is associated with an increased risk of birth defects, particularly neural tube defects such as spina bifida.

- Obesity in premenopausal women is associated with irregular menstrual cycles and infertility.

◆ Additional Health Concerns
  - Overweight and obesity are associated with increased risks of gallbladder disease, stress incontinence (urine leakage from weak pelvic floor muscles), increased surgical risk, and depression.

  - Obesity can affect the quality of life through limited mobility and decreased physical endurance.

Your Story

"I have tried everything else."
"I am destined to be overweight."
"There is no use to try anymore."
This is not true. You do not have to be overweight or obese. Even if you have struggled with your weight your whole life. Even if you have tried everything else, only to be let down.

My daughter and I wrote this book for Black women because of the overwhelming amount of misinformation that exists on what it takes for Black women to reach and maintain a healthy weight. The *Weight Loss Programs*, *Weight Loss Strategies*, and *Maintenance Program* in this book are based on my 30+ years of experience in studying, researching, listening to, counseling, and personally treating thousands of Black women for weight loss as a medical doctor.

This is a real weight loss solution for Black women because it takes into account the physiology, psychology, and sociology of Black women.

"I spend my life taking care of others."
"I do not have time to diet."
"I have no will power to diet."

You are making a choice about your life. Even though you spend much time on your children, your spouse, your parents, your education, your career, and your church activities, you must take care of yourself.

There are too many bad health consequences of obesity including premature death, heart disease, stroke, diabetes, cancer, breathing problems, arthritis, and reproductive complications to ignore it. Those who depend on you will be much worse off if you are not around or not able to take care of them. If it is just you, it will be much worse on you personally to have to deal with a preventable disease rather than being healthy.

Will power and an abundance of time are not necessary. The *Weight Loss Strategies* in Chapter 4 offer suggestions on how to deal with life's daily challenges as you are on your journey to a healthy weight. The *Recipes* in Appendix B contain easy-to-prepare meals with all of the foods on the *Weight Loss Programs*.

"I am only 20 pounds overweight, it is not that serious."

All seriously overweight women began only a few pounds overweight. It is never too early to stop obesity's natural progression. Remember, you do not have to do anything wrong to gain weight. It is based on your genetic makeup. Your weight gain is naturally occurring.

The earlier you start, the greater the chance you will have at not becoming obese. This will go a long way in reducing the risk of obesity-related health consequences including premature death, heart disease, stroke, diabetes, cancer, breathing problems, arthritis, and reproductive complications.

As you get older, it becomes more difficult to lose weight. Also, as you get older, extra weight is a much greater strain on your heart, respiratory system, and bones. Start losing weight now!

If you have children, please read the section on *Children and the Weight Loss Program* in Chapter 3 *Weight Loss Programs*.

"I have been eating healthy, but I still cannot reach my goal weight."

If you have been *eating healthy* in order to lose weight, you may have found that you lost some weight, but that you reached a plateau fairly quickly. If you started at 205 pounds, ate healthy, started exercising, lost 15 pounds, but now cannot get past a weight of 190 pounds, that means your body "naturally" wants to weigh 190 pounds.

You have already given up pancakes, fried eggs, cheese grits, and bacon for breakfast; hamburgers and French fries for lunch; fried pork chops, macaroni and cheese, candied yams, and biscuits for dinner; ice cream for dessert; and candy bars and chips for snacks all day long. That may have been quite an accomplishment.

But, while having an egg white, bagel, and orange juice for breakfast; a lean roast beef sandwich on wheat bread for lunch; turkey wings, brown rice, corn, and a small dinner roll for dinner; yogurt for dessert; and granola bars for snacks is very healthy eating, you will not lose weight. You are not overeating, and you are not eating anything too fattening. Essentially, you are giving your body what it needs and nothing more, so you will not rapidly gain weight. However, you will not lose all of your excess weight.

You have to first force your body into the unnatural act of "eating to lose" by following the *Weight Loss Programs* covered in Chapter 3. That is the only way you will get to a healthy weight. None of the foods mentioned above will force your body to use your fat as a source of energy. You will not lose all of your excess weight eating those foods. None of the foods mentioned above is on the *Weight Loss Programs*.

Once you reach a healthy weight, then you will be "eating to maintain," or essentially eating healthy by following the *Maintenance Program* covered in Chapter 5. Once you are at your goal, you will be able to eat your favorite foods in moderation.

"I lost weight and was happy, but now I have gained it all back, plus some."

This is a Two-Step process. If you lost weight, but did not go on a maintenance program, then your body grew back to its "natural" state. The same thing would happen to your hair if you did not have and implement a maintenance program.

Your body also changes as you get older, or have the first baby, or have the second baby, or reach menopause, or have gynecological surgery. None of our bodies is the same as they were five years ago.

You must follow the *Weight Loss Programs* in Chapter 3 to lose weight, then you must follow the *Maintenance Program* in Chapter 5 to maintain a healthy weight for the rest of your life.

"I am on so many medications and have so many ailments that I will not be able to follow the weight loss program."

Losing as little as 10 pounds can reduce the effects and symptoms of many diseases and ailments. Share this book with your physician. By working together and using the guidelines in this book, you will be able to develop a plan to help you lose weight in conjunction with your other medications and treatment.

"I am overweight and I love who I am. There is no need for me to be thin."

Loving yourself, no matter what, is a wonderful thing, especially if you reached that point after a lifetime of emotional, family, financial, and educational challenges. Getting to a healthy weight is not about being thin, it is not about being a "single-digit woman."

The primary concern of obesity is one of health and not one of appearance. There are too many health consequences including premature death, heart disease, stroke, diabetes, cancer, breathing problems, arthritis, and reproductive complications to remain obese.

Once your weight is in the *Healthy Range*, how small you go from there is strictly a personal decision. You do not have to be thin, but you must get to and maintain a healthy weight.

"My man does not like skinny women."

It is probably safe to say that we Black men generally do not prefer skinny women. It is a matter of personal and cultural preference. Also, we do not want to see our women suffer, and we may equate dieting with suffering.

However, we do love our women. Therefore, you must convince your Black man that you are losing weight *only* for health reasons. We do not want you to be in bad health. If we think that you are dieting only for looks and we like the way you look as you are, then we are not likely to aid and support the weight loss program.

Reaching a healthy weight does not have to be about being skinny. It does not have to be about "trying to be cute." The primary concern of obesity is one of health and not one of appearance. Please ask your spouse to read Appendix A *A Note to Your Spouse*.

"I would lose weight if I would just exercise."
"I do exercise, but I am not losing weight."

You cannot simply exercise weight off of Black women. Exercise is good for the cardiovascular system, it helps with toning the muscles, it helps flexibility, it helps with the *Maintenance Program*, and it helps you feel better. However, heavy exercise–including running, lifting weights, squats, stair climbing, high impact aerobics, and riding a bicycle–will not help you lose weight. In fact, if you are overweight or obese, these activities can be very dangerous.

You will build muscle, and yes, muscle does weigh more than fat. You may be "in shape," but if you weigh over 170 pounds at 5'6", your risk for serious obesity-related health consequences still exists, especially as you get older or can no longer maintain a strict and rigorous exercise regimen.

You may also notice from heavy exercise that you are getting bigger instead of getting smaller. Heavy lower body exercises will increase hip and thigh muscle bulk and will make hips and thighs larger in the long run. In other words, you will be getting bulkier instead of slimmer.

Think about the slaves who used to work in the fields. Now that was some exercise. There was bending, lifting, sweating, and the burning of many calories. Those were usually not small women.

The *Weight Loss Programs* in Chapter 3 include the correct and safe exercise regimens for getting to a healthy weight.

"My man has me on the same diet and exercise program that he is on, but I am not losing weight."

The body of your man is totally different from your body. He can hit the gym for one hour a few days a week, cut out the fried food, and lose weight quickly. You follow the same program that he does, but you do not lose weight.

The key physiological difference between men and women relates to the fact that the male hormone, testosterone, is a much more potent energy-using hormone than the female hormone, estrogen. Men tend to have larger, stronger muscles and less subcutaneous fat than women, which means they have a higher metabolic rate and their bodies burn more calories throughout the day than women.

Please ask him to read Appendix A *A Note to Your Spouse* in Appendix A.

"My sister can eat whatever she wants and not gain weight. Why do I have to struggle with my weight?"

Have you ever seen a litter of puppies? There is always a runt and there is always a big guy. Even with the same parents, each offspring is different. In addition, you and your sister's differing ages, number of children, and previous illnesses can play a significant role. Your sister may have it easier in the weight department, but I am sure that you were born with some things she wishes she had.

"I was not overweight until I turned 30 years old."
"I was not overweight until I had a baby."
"I was not overweight until I got on birth control."
Some inherited characteristics in humans are not present at birth, but show up only when they are triggered by an event. The example we all know is gray hair. It is usually not present at birth even though it is inherited. It is triggered by age.

If your father had the genes for gray hair and your mother had the genes for gray hair, and both died at the age of 25, then you may not know that they had the genes. You may get gray hair if you live long enough to trigger it.

Obesity may be present at birth, or it may be triggered by age, or it may be triggered by childbirth number 1, or it may be triggered by childbirth number 2, or it may be triggered by taking hormones, or it may be triggered by menopause, or it may be triggered by a hysterectomy, etc.

Regardless of what may have triggered your weight gain, the *Weight Loss Programs* in Chapter 3 will get you to a healthy weight, and the *Maintenance Program* in Chapter 5 will allow you to stay at a healthy weight for the rest of your life.

"I want to be a single-digit woman – so what?"

You do not have to make excuses about wanting to be thin. You may like the way your clothes fit when you are a size 6. Your career may dictate that you are on the small side. You may want to look like a strong, toned, and muscular woman at age 50. Your goal weight is your own personal decision. Do not let anyone get you off track based on his or her own prejudices, jealousies, and controlling ways.

For Religious Leaders

As the Reverend, First Lady, Deaconess, or other leader of your church you may be constantly faced with members offering you food. In addition, there are many functions you must attend in an official capacity such as church socials, cookouts, banquets, wedding receptions, and funeral repasses.

However, as a religious leader, you obviously realize that the health of your congregation is one of your responsibilities. You should lead by example by maintaining a healthy weight for yourself and your family, and by emphasizing the dangers of obesity in our people.

Remember that you are being given food out of love and respect. It is difficult, but it is your responsibility to reject the food *without* rejecting the love and respect of the giver. You do this by being proactive. Let your members know that you are encouraging healthy weight and nutrition.

You can promote a healthy weight loss program in association with a physician in your congregation. If there are none, then you can approach your personal physician to oversee the weight loss program in your members.

Two

WEIGHT LOSS FUNDAMENTALS

Body Composition and Weight

The body is composed of different components – fat tissue, lean tissue, organ tissue, bones, and fluids – each having a different weight and density. The body appears to have a solid sameness from day to day; however, the particles that make up the organs and tissues are in a constant state of flux. The continuous exchange of particles in the tissues accounts for the continuous changes in weight.

Large factors – like temporary retention of water in the body, food in the stomach, the amount of water lost through perspiration, kidney functions, and intestinal functions – can make your body weight, as measured on the bathroom scale, vary each day. The scale may even show a different weight in the late afternoon than it did in the morning.

For this reason, I recommend weighing yourself only once a week at the same time of day. Although your caloric intake will be reduced, given the fact that your body is in a constant state of flux, weight loss may not be reflected immediately. The different turnover rates of the body pause at each new level of lower body weight before descending to the next lower weight level.

Fat Cells

The fat mass is composed of essential fat and storage fat. The essential fat is a required component of the brain, nerves, bone marrow, heart tissue, and cell walls that you cannot live without. Adult females also have a large part of their essential fat as breast tissue. Obesity results when the size and number of fat cells in a person's body increase. A normal-sized person has between 30 and 35 billion fat cells. When a person gains weight, these fat cells increase first in size and later in number.

One pound of body fat has approximately 3,500 calories of stored energy. When a person starts losing weight, the cells decrease in size, but it is thought that the number of fat cells generally stays the same. This is part of the reason that once you lose and regain a significant amount of weight, it is more difficult to lose it again.

Metabolism

Metabolism is the act or process by which living tissues or cells take up and convert into their own proper substance the nutritive material brought to them by the blood, or by which they transform their cell protoplasm into simpler substances which are fitted either for excretion or for some special purpose, as in the manufacture of the digestive ferments. It includes all physical and chemical processes within the body related to the generation and use of energy for nutrition, digestion, absorption, elimination, respiration, circulation, and temperature regulation.

In very simple terms, your metabolism is the rate at which your individual body engine operates as it performs all its bodily functions, like the creation and building of various substances (proteins, muscle, enzymes, nails, storage fat, hair, bones), the breaking down of others (storage fat, food), and the production of heat. Both the creation and building process (anabolic) and the breaking down process (catabolic) occur constantly and at the same time. The fuel for all the chemical reactions that make up the metabolic process is the nutrients contained in food.

Women who have a difficult time losing weight often think that they have a "slow metabolism" and want to speed it up so they can lose more. The term "metabolism" and the term "metabolic rate" are used interchangeably. The metabolic rate is sped up noticeably with aerobic exercise. When you finish an aerobic workout, your metabolic rate is much higher than at other times, but think about how you are feeling then. You are breathing fast, your heart is beating fast, you are sweating, and your blood pressure may be up.

This is not a safe state that you would want to be in all the time. So while it is possible to speed up your metabolism, it is not safe or wise. Certain misguided or unscrupulous individuals would have you believe that certain drugs such as thyroid or ephedra or other "metabolic enhancers" will speed up your metabolism and increase the rate of weight loss. Those agents *do not* speed up the metabolism and they are not safe.

Thyroid Problems

It is rare that a person is overweight because of an underactive thyroid gland. There is a specific test, the serum thyroid stimulating hormone level, which will determine whether or not you have an underactive thyroid. If the test is high, you have an underactive thyroid. If it is normal, you do not. It is as simple as that.

Certain "herbologists," and even certain physicians, will give synthetic or natural thyroid hormone pills or capsules to a person who either has not been tested or who has normal tests in the mistaken belief that this will accelerate weight loss. This is dangerous, unhealthy, and wrong. Do not ever take synthetic or natural thyroid in an attempt to lose weight if you do not have an abnormally high serum thyroid stimulating hormone level.

The Importance of Water

Considering that your body is almost two-thirds water, understanding water's important role in the body can be a fountain of health. Next to oxygen, water is the human body's most important substance. It plays a vital role in regulating body temperature, transporting nutrients and oxygen to cells, removing waste and toxins, cushioning joints, and protecting organs and tissues. Water is even needed to breathe. Your lungs must be moistened by water in order to effectively take in oxygen and get rid of carbon dioxide. You lose approximately a pint of liquid each day exhaling.

The ability of water to dissolve a multitude of substances allows your cells to utilize valuable nutrients, minerals, and chemicals in biological processes, and water's surface tension enables your body to mobilize these elements efficiently. Water helps your body digest food more efficiently, suppresses the appetite naturally, and helps your body metabolize stored fat. Your body loses water via the skin by perspiration, via the kidneys by urine, via the lungs by exhaled water vapor, and via the intestine by feces.

Especially while you are following your *Weight Loss Program*, if you do not drink enough water then your body will metabolize the fat slower. You may retain fluid and that will cause the scale to go up. Dark-colored urine may suggest that you are not drinking enough water.

Drinking enough water may be the best treatment for fluid retention. When the body gets less water, it perceives this as a threat to survival and begins to hold on to every drop. Water is stored in spaces inside and outside the cells. This may show up as swollen feet and legs. Strange as it may seem, one of the ways to eliminate fluid retention is to drink more water, not less.

Drink Your Water

You must drink two to three quarts of water per day. This is at least eight glasses of water with each glass containing eight ounces.

◆ Drink one extra glass of water for each 30 minutes of exercise.

◆ Drink one extra glass of water for each cup of coffee or black tea you consume.

◆ If you have inhalant allergies, drink as much water as possible, especially during the major allergy seasons.

What type of water is best?

You may use activated carbon or charcoal filters on your faucet to inexpensively remove the carcinogens and bacteria commonly found in tap water. With bottled water, verify that your brand has been tested for bacterial and chemical levels.

Do not drink flavored water (even if the package says "no calories") or seltzer water as I have found over the years that drinking these types of water do not help you lose weight. The chemicals that give the water flavor may cause fluid retention.

Other Benefits of Drinking Water

◆ Drinking water can help reduce daytime fatigue.

◆ Drinking one glass of water an hour before going to bed can help reduce midnight hunger pangs.

◆ Even mild dehydration may slow down your metabolism as much as 3%.

◆ As you are following your *Weight Loss Program*, water helps to flush out the body.

◆ Preliminary research indicates that drinking two to three quarts of water per day may significantly ease joint and back pain.

Diuretics, Fluid Retention, and Sodium

Diuretics work within the kidneys to increase the excretion of excess fluid and sodium from the body. They are sometimes known as "fluid pills" or "water pills." For many people, diuretics are a lifesaver. The pathological buildup of fluids in the lungs, the abdomen, and the lower legs is enough to cause serious breathing and functional changes in the body, sometimes enough to cause death.

Diuretics are also useful for the person with hypertension (high blood pressure) because they can lower the amount of excess fluid in the body, thereby causing the blood pressure to drop. In cases of overuse, however, the loss of too much fluid and sodium causes weakness. This is similar to the symptoms of heat exhaustion from losing too much fluid and sodium through sweating. The person who abuses these diuretics finds herself with weakness, muscle spasms and cramping, and a shortage of two other vital minerals – potassium and magnesium.

Dieters also tend to collect unwanted fluid and sodium. The discomfort of fluid retention can be relieved by intelligent use of diuretics. For dieters, the ideal way to take these medications is once every two to four nights. Because there is a 48- to 72- hour interval between doses, the body has a chance to recoup the losses of minerals other than sodium. Night is the best time to take the diuretics, when the body is lying flat and fluid pooled in the lower part of the body has a chance, through gravity, to equalize and make more sodium available to the kidneys to be filtered out.

It is estimated that almost twice as much fluid and sodium can be gotten rid of if diuretics are taken at night. It is true that getting up at night is a problem for some people, but the increased efficiency of action is worth it!

Drinking large amounts of water during the day and just before retiring is an excellent way to "prime the pump" and increase fluid and sodium loss. The extra water makes the sodium loss much greater and helps carry out other waste products that accumulate whenever a large amount of fat is lost.

Do not take diuretics except under the care of your physician. Only take diuretics as prescribed.

Carbohydrates

Carbohydrates are divided into two types–simple and complex. The simple carbohydrates are mostly referred to as sugars. They are the monosaccharides (fructose, galactose, and glucose), disaccharides (sucrose, lactose, and maltose), and the rare oligosaccharides (fructans). The complex carbohydrates are mostly referred to as starches. They are the polysaccharides, or plant starches, such as cellulose, gums, and pectin. All carbohydrates are a good source of energy, but the starches provide a better source of long-term energy.

Starches including rice, pasta, potatoes, beans, bread and crackers, actually help save the body fat in times of insufficient caloric intake. That is why grains are given to starving people in underdeveloped countries. A person can live for a long time on grain alone. However, when you are trying to lose weight, you do not want a good source of long-term energy. You want your body to use its stored fat as a source of energy.

For weight reduction purposes, I have found that starches are not necessary to maintain good health. In fact, they slow the rate of weight loss. This is why there are no starches on our *Weight Loss Programs*. Fruits and vegetables are absolutely necessary, however, to maintain good health while dieting.

Dietary Fats

There are three types of dietary fats–saturated fats, unsaturated fats, and essential fatty acids. Fats are necessary for good health, however, an excessive amount of saturated fats is dangerous.

Saturated fats are those found in red meat, cheese, butter, sour cream, and coconut oils.

Unsaturated fats are usually liquid at room temperature. They are found in most vegetable products and oils. An exception is a group of tropical oils like coconut or palm kernel oil which is highly saturated. Using foods containing "polyunsaturated" and "monounsaturated" fats does not significantly increase your risk of heart disease. However, like all fats, unsaturated fats give us about nine calories for every gram. Eating too much of these types of fats may also make you gain weight.

Essential fatty acids cannot be synthesized by the body, but are essential for good health. They aid in the production of hemoglobin; increase resistance to viruses and bacteria; assist the functions of glands and hormones; nourish the skin, hair, and nails; lower high blood pressure; lower triglyceride levels; aid in the eradication of plaque from the arterial walls; increase the rate at which the body burns fat; and perform many other functions too numerous to list for our purposes here.

The essential fatty acids are linoleic acid, linolenic acid, and arachidonic acid. Linoleic acid can be converted by the body into linlolenic or arachidonic, but linoleic acid must be eaten. Good sources of essential fatty acids are cold water fish oils such as sardines, cod, tuna, salmon, herring, and mackerel; natural soybean oil; wheat-germ oil; dried beans; safflower oils; sunflower oils; and corn oils.

There is a "hybrid" of fats called trans fats, created through a man-made process developed in late nineteenth-century Germany. Trans fats are produced through hydrogenation, a chemical process by which hydrogen is added to unsaturated fatty acids. Hydrogenation converts the unsaturated bonds in the oil into saturated bonds, creating a solid, spreadable fat, that increases the shelf life and flavor of foods.

Research analyzed by the Food and Drug Administration indicates that trans fats raise blood cholesterol levels–in particular LDL, "bad cholesterol," which increase the risk of coronary heart disease. Trans fats also reduce HDL, "good cholesterol," and increase triglycerides. Reduced HDL and high triglycerides are associated with insulin resistance. At the National Obesity and Weight Control Symposium in New York in April 1993, it was reported that increases in dietary trans fatty acids affect muscle membranes in a manner that could trigger diabetes and could be worsened if the person is obese.

Trans fats are found in foods such as vegetable shortening, some margarines, crackers, candies, baked goods, fried foods, cookies, snack foods, many processed foods, and the oil used for deep frying in fast food restaurants.

By January 1, 2006 the nutritional facts labels on foods and dietary supplements must contain a line that lists the amount of trans fat in the product. Until then, read the labels. If you see the words "hydrogenated" or "partially hydrogenated" in front of any vegetable oil, the food contains trans fats.

Remember that an excessive amount of all these fats will decrease the rate of weight loss. It is important to follow the directions of the *Weight Loss Programs* in Chapter 3 in order to lose weight while getting all of the essential fatty acids.

Vegetarianism

Many think that because a vegetarian diet is low in saturated fats, it is healthy and promotes weight loss. The first part of this is true. A vegetarian diet can be healthy. However, a vegetarian diet must have a source of protein to be healthy. The main sources of non-animal protein are beans, but protein is also found in other parts of the plant.

Beans, though, are also high in starch and, as said before, starches save the body fat. Therefore, a diet containing beans or bean products such as tofu and veggie burgers will not allow most overweight and obese Black women to lose weight.

If you are a vegan and want to lose weight, you must intake your protein in the form of protein drinks which contain mostly plant protein without the starch or sugars. You must read the label. It is dangerous to attempt to lose a significant amount of weight without adequate protein intake.

Hips and Thighs
Stretch Marks
Cellulite

Unfortunately, there are no proven, effective, non-surgical, permanent methods for spot reducing hips or thighs, or for removing stretch marks, or for removing cellulite.

If you are essentially satisfied with your weight, but your hips and thighs are what you consider to be "out of proportion," liposuction *may* help.

If you have abdominal stretch marks secondary to pregnancy or because you have had a large abdomen for many years, the surgical "tummy tuck" may be your only option for making them less visible.

None of the anti-cellulite creams, lotions, and potions has been proven to work permanently or consistently. Again, liposuction seems to be the only treatment.

Obesity, Pregnancy, and Dieting

It is risky to get pregnant when you are overweight and obese. The best scenario is to lose the weight, maintain the loss for two to three months, and then get pregnant.

As you lose weight, you become more fertile. If you are not interested in getting pregnant, make sure you implement a birth control plan. I have treated many patients who were told that they could not get pregnant, only to get pregnant after losing as few as 20 pounds.

If you do get pregnant, cease your *Weight Loss Program* immediately, as it is very dangerous for your unborn child. When you are on a weight reduction diet, you are forcing your body to live partly on its own tissue; fat is a living tissue. That is abnormal physiology. Normally you do not live on your own tissue. Normally you live on food.

When you are pregnant, your main function is to provide a healthy environment for the developing baby. Therefore, you should be living normally, with good healthy food, vitamins, minerals, and milk if you can digest it. It is especially dangerous to take diet pills during pregnancy because we do not know for a fact what harm diet pills can do to the developing baby.

Losing Weight After Pregnancy

When you are pregnant, especially in the later stages, your body stores fat in preparation for producing milk for the newborn. Many calories are required to produce milk, and the body does not rely on your eating enough food to produce milk at the time the baby will need it. It has been stated that the human can breast-feed for six to eight months. If you do not breast-feed at all or if you do not breast-feed for that period of time, the fat stays on your body. While there is no hard scientific proof, it seems as though this fat is harder to lose than the fat produced in the non-pregnant state. Nevertheless, the procedures for losing weight are the same.

Losing Weight After Menopause and Gynecological Surgery

Pre-menopause, menopause, a hysterectomy, and any other type of gynecological surgery often seem to make it harder to lose weight. The reasons have not been investigated sufficiently for us to know exactly why this occurs, but the procedures for losing weight are the same as in other cases.

Weight Loss Myths

Since there is so much misinformation on how to lose weight safely and effectively, it is important to understand why many of these methods, pills, and supplements do not work and, in some cases, may be harmful.

Low Carb Diets

The typical low carb or no carb diet is dangerous. The proponents of low carb diets often do not stress the fact that fruits and vegetables are necessary for good health while losing weight. They should only be emphasizing the omission of starches from the weight loss diet, not the elimination of fruits and vegetables.

All of our *Weight Loss Programs* include ample fruits and vegetables. The National Cancer Institute states that the risk of cancer increases when most fruits and vegetables are eliminated from the diet. Low carb, low fiber diets are high in animal protein, saturated fat, and cholesterol, increasing the risk of heart disease. These also raise the LDL "bad cholesterol". Kidney stones, gout, and osteoporosis are also more likely to occur in high protein, low carb diets.

Eating Just a Little Bit of Food

Common sense states that "the less you eat, the faster you lose." However, common sense is usually wrong in this case, especially if you have over 10 pounds to lose and want the weight to stay off. Common sense does not take into account the fact that if you eat too small an amount of calories, the body will respond by slowing the metabolism and burning significant amounts of lean body tissue as a source of fuel or energy. That is not safe and is counter-productive.

You must intake the correct type and amount of food for your body weight in order to keep the metabolic rate high enough to burn mostly fat. Chapter 3 *Weight Loss Programs* outlines how much you must eat in order to lose safely as determined by your present body weight.

Fasting to Lose Weight

Different religious practices call for periodic fasts to spiritually cleanse the body and soul. But, can a non-religiously-based 24- to 48- hour fast, with or without juices or other fluids, lead to a physical cleansing? No.

A fast that lasts more than a couple of days can actually impede the body's efforts to keep its insides clean. To conserve energy during what it perceives as a period of starvation, the body undergoes a slowdown of all its functions, including the processes in the liver and other organs that detoxify or eliminate potentially harmful chemicals.

Granted, some people say they feel better after a fast, even if it does cause fatigue, dizziness, irritability, or depression. As long as the fast does not last more than 24 to 48 hours, it will not do any real harm.

The positive response to fasting is psychological rather than physiological. Fasting might help you reach a state of spiritual cleanliness, or it may just make you feel like you have beaten hunger at its own game, if only for a short period of time.

Body Wraps

Body wraps and herbal wraps are often marketed as a method of losing inches and weight rapidly. In fact, these chemical wraps dehydrate the subcutaneous tissue and cause you to temporarily lose inches. Even though the number on the scale may go down, this is not a true loss of fat; it is a loss of water.

If that is what you want and you are in otherwise good health, these wraps are not usually harmful. If you are on *any* medication, ask your physician before you let anyone wrap you in these chemically impregnated materials.

Using Diuretics to Lose Weight

Many people are under the impression that taking diuretics or water pills helps their weight loss. Nothing could be further from the truth. The only thing that diuretics do in the normal obese patient is to remove water, along with sometimes badly needed minerals, from the body. The loss of these minerals, such as potassium and magnesium, can cause weakness, muscle spasms, and even severe illness in some patients. During your menstrual period you may notice that you are retaining fluid, but a high water intake is superior to diuretics in getting rid of excess and unwanted water bloating.

Only take diuretics under the supervision of your physician. Use them as intended and they will help. If your feet and ankles are not swollen at the end of the day or if you do not have hypertension, do not use them. Never get diuretics from a non-physician or over the Internet.

Three

WEIGHT LOSS PROGRAMS

The *Weight Loss Programs* contain "weight losing diets." These are not diets to follow for the rest of your life. You will be "eating to lose," not "eating to maintain."

Once you reach your goal, you must follow the *Maintenance Program* covered in Chapter 5 to maintain your healthy weight.

Select the **Weight Loss Program** based on how much you presently weigh:

- **Weight Loss Program A** – Over 230 pounds

- **Weight Loss Program B** – 191 pounds to 230 pounds

- **Weight Loss Program C** – 160 pounds to 190 pounds

- **Weight Loss Program D** – Under 160 pounds

The meals, allowed foods, snacks, and exercise plans are described individually and in a separate section for each *Weight Loss Program*. Follow only the *Weight Loss Program* for your present weight; otherwise you will not get the desired results and it could be dangerous.

For example, if you are 150 pounds and follow *Weight Loss Program C*, then you will not lose weight. If you are 220 pounds and follow *Weight Loss Program D*, then you may get sick.

Men and the Weight Loss Programs

Men usually lose weight faster than women because testosterone is a far more efficient fat-burning aid than estrogen. Men who have more than 10 pounds of excess weight should follow only *Weight Loss Program A*. Men who have less than 10 pounds of excess weight should follow only *Weight Loss Program B*.

Men should never follow *Weight Loss Program C* or *Weight Loss Program D* because there are too few calories to make the program safe and effective.

Children and the Weight Loss Programs

Overweight children are especially difficult to treat. Most obese children are overweight due to a combination of excess caloric intake and heredity. However, simply trying to reduce the caloric intake and increase exercise usually does not produce satisfactory results. The child may see caloric restriction as a form of suffering or punishment and will not cooperate.

Often a family member or friend does not recognize obesity as a health problem and "sneaks" food to the child. In addition, there is the danger of interfering with normal growth and development when you are trying to force the developing body to use its own tissue (fat is a living tissue) as a source of energy or fuel.

Do not have a child follow the *Weight Loss Programs* in this book.

If you have an overweight child under the age of 15, you must have the child in an organized weight control program under the supervision of experienced physicians. Talk to your child's pediatrician or contact the American Society of Bariatric Physicians on the Web at www.asbp.org or by phone at 303-770-2526.

Before Getting Started

1. If you have hypertension or heart disease.
When you have uncontrolled hypertension or heart disease, you are at risk if you increase the stress on your heart or blood vessels. Exercise temporarily increases the blood pressure. Avoid exercise if you have uncontrolled hypertension or heart disease.

If your hypertension and heart disease are controlled by medication, the interaction of your medication and appetite suppressants can be problematic. Also, you may be on diuretics. Rapid weight loss involves the loss of some fluid. This is unavoidable and even desirable. However, the loss of fluid often leads to the loss of necessary body potassium. You should get the proper replacement potassium supplements.

Do not start on the *Weight Loss Program* until you talk to your physician. He or she will advise you as to what is safe and what is dangerous. If your physician will not help you, seek the assistance of a bariatric physician.

2. If you have diabetes.
In the normal, non-diabetic person, the body produces the correct amount of insulin to maintain the blood sugar at a healthy level, based on what the person eats or has eaten. In the diabetic, the body either produces no insulin or produces an insufficient amount to maintain the blood sugar at the normal level. Hence, in the treatment of diabetes, the person is given insulin or oral medications in order to allow the body to maintain the correct level.

However, that level of medication is usually given in a set amount at a certain time each day. It is not given in response to what the person just ate. Therefore, when you lower what you eat or lower your weight, the amount of medication that was correct will become too much and your sugar can drop too low.

The goal of weight loss in diabetics is to lower or stop the need for antidiabetic medications. Therefore, the medications must be carefully monitored with an eye on the blood sugar so that the level will not drop too low. As the blood sugar drops, the antidiabetic medication must be dropped also.

Most diabetics monitor their own blood sugar on a daily basis. If your blood sugar drops below 100 units, notify your physician immediately.

Do not start on the *Weight Loss Program* until you talk to your physician. He or she will advise you as to what is safe and what is dangerous. If your physician will not help you, then seek the assistance of a bariatric physician.

3. If you are pregnant.

When you are pregnant, your major concern is in providing the optimum environment for the unborn baby. Hence, you should not be living on your own tissue (fat) or putting medications (diet pills) in your bloodstream.

Do not follow the *Weight Loss Program* while you are pregnant. Follow your obstetrician's instructions, get good prenatal care, and avoid the manufacture of unnecessary new fat.

Once you have finished breast-feeding, then you may start following the *Weight Loss Program*.

4. If you want to get pregnant.

As you lose weight, you will become more fertile. It is not uncommon for a woman to lose just 20 pounds and get pregnant, even if she had been told that she was unable to get pregnant.

While you are on the *Weight Loss Program*, use a birth control method. Cease with the *Weight Loss Program* when you are trying to conceive.

5. If you take medications that require eating food.

The purpose of eating food or drinking milk with medication is to avoid nausea and/or damage to the stomach lining if the medication remains in the stomach too long. To facilitate this, take the medication with a can of tuna, not bread, and drink 10 ounces of water.

Expected Results

Unless instructed by your physician, combining this *Weight Loss Program* with any other food lists, eating plans, meal replacements, exercise regimens, and diet supplements that you have heard about or tried will not help you lose weight. If you combine this program with other methods, you will not reach and maintain a healthy weight.

How Much Weight Should You Lose?

Following the *Weight Loss Program*, you can expect to lose between 8 to 15 pounds per month depending on your present weight. The more you weigh, the more in actual pounds you will lose. As you lose weight, you may notice that while you used to lose 13 pounds per month, you are now only losing 11 pounds per month. This is because there are fewer total pounds than before.

Here is an example. If you started at a weight of 225 pounds and lost 13 pounds in one month, that would be a weight loss percentage of approximately 5.8% (13 divided by 225). Now at 190 pounds you are losing 11 pounds per month, but that is still a weight loss percentage of approximately 5.8% (11 divided by 190) as well. Therefore, you are staying on track and consistently losing weight. At a weight of 160 pounds, 5.8% is equivalent to just over 9 pounds. At a weight of 270 pounds, 5.8% is equivalent to just over 15 pounds.

When to Weigh Yourself

Pick one day per week to weigh yourself. You will weigh yourself when you first arise for your day, in the nude and with an empty bladder. A suggestion is to weigh yourself mid-week, such as every Wednesday morning. Your weight should be obtained using a good bathroom scale. Avoid cheap digital scales as they are too unreliable. Do not let anyone change the settings on your scale for any reason.

Keep a weekly record of your weight. Plotting your weight on a graph gives you a good visual indication of your progress.

Try not to weigh yourself every day and especially try not to weigh yourself multiple times during the day. Your weight varies slightly during the day based on several conditions including the last time you ate, the last time you went to the bathroom, and how much liquid you have consumed.

You can become disappointed very quickly if you weigh yourself every day or several times during the day. The number on the scale erroneously becomes a gauge of how well you have done your *Weight Loss Program* that day. You know that you have followed your *Weight Loss Program*, but the scale is the same as yesterday or, even more disastrous, it has gone up. You believe the scale and not your actions. This kind of disappointment can easily cause you to go off your *Weight Loss Program*. Remember that the scale does not just measure fat; it also measures weight, which includes water weight, lean body tissue, and bowel contents.

Your Body Is on a 28-Day Cycle

While you will weigh yourself every seven days, your body is not on a seven-day cycle. Your body is actually on a 28-day cycle. You will see that at different times of the month, your weight loss varies. Some women retain fluid at various times during the month. Fluid retention may happen before, during, or after your period. Even if you no longer have a period, you may notice fluid retention at certain times of the month. Fluid retention is most often recognized by the tightness of the rings on your fingers or the snugness of the shoes on your feet.

Therefore, do not expect to lose the exact same amount of weight each week. You may have a four-pound loss week, then a two-pound loss week, then a three-pound loss week.

Even when the scale goes down only a pound or two, you may notice that you are losing inches. This is another indication that the *Weight Loss Program* is working. Stay on your *Weight Loss Program* and the pounds on the scale will catch up.

Your success on the *Weight Loss Program* is measured by the trend of your weight loss. As long as you are consistently losing between 8 to 15 pounds on a month-to-month basis, stay on track with your current *Weight Loss Program*.

Recipes

We have included many recipes in *Appendix B*. This list of recipes is by no means exhaustive. You may create your meals as you desire, as long as they contain only the foods on your *Weight Loss Program*.

Food Preparation

Foods may be eaten raw, baked, broiled, grilled, blackened, or boiled *without* oil, butter, margarine, or fats of any kind.

You may use the following to prepare your food:

- ◆ Fat-free cooking spray

- ◆ Any spices including garlic powder, salt, pepper, and onion powder. There are many wonderful spice blends such as lemon pepper, garlic and herb, and Mrs. Dash®. Visit the spice section in the grocery store for additional ideas on how to spice up your food.

- ◆ Fat-free mayonnaise

- ◆ Fat-free salad dressing

- ◆ Lemon (fresh or lemon drops)

- Mustard

- Equal®, Splenda®, or NutraSweet®

- Vinegar

- Garlic

You *may not* use the following to prepare your food because they may contain too many calories or too much sugar, sodium, and/or fat:

- Marinades

- Anything that ends in the word "sauce"–soy sauce, BBQ sauce, honey mustard sauce, tartar sauce, cocktail sauce, teriyaki sauce, sweet and sour sauce, etc.

- Oil, butter, margarine, or fats of any kind

- Bouillon

- Turkey wings, thighs, legs, or necks

- Pork

- Wine or cooking sherry

Juicing

Juicing fruits and vegetables is not recommended. The body requires a certain amount of energy (calories) to digest fruits and vegetables. This "work" aids in weight loss. Once "juiced," the body does not require nearly the same amount of energy for digestion.

Juicing makes the sugar too readily available to the system and slows the burning of stored fat. In addition, it requires eating a greater amount of fruits and vegetables to make just one glass of juice. This increases your caloric intake. For example, compare the number of oranges you would use to make one glass of juice versus the number of oranges you would eat in one sitting.

Foods and Drinks That Are Not Allowed

Do not eat or drink anything that is not listed on your *Weight Loss Program*. From our experience in treating thousands of Black women for weight loss, we have found that these foods do not help you lose weight.

While many of these foods may be considered "healthy" or "good for you," and may not make you gain weight, the purpose of the *Weight Loss Program* is to lose weight. Eating "healthy" will enable you to maintain your weight.

Once you are on the *Maintenance Program*, you may be able to eat these foods in moderation. Many of these foods are high in calories, sugars, sodium and/or fats.

Do Not Eat:

◆ **Starches**– (rice, pasta, potatoes, bread, beans, crackers)– starches help to store body fat. See the section on *Carbohydrates* in Chapter 2.

◆ **Soup**– may be high in sodium and may also contain items that are not on the *Weight Loss Program*.

◆ **Nuts**– high in calories and fat.

◆ **Juice**– high in calories and sugars; in addition, drinking juice may make you hungry later.

◆ **Dairy** (whole milk, skim milk, cheese, cream, yogurt)– may be high in calories and fat; in addition, drinking milk is necessary only for growing children and mothers who are breast-feeding. See the section on *Supplements* later in this chapter.

Do Not Eat (cont.)

- **Cereal**– may be high in calories, fat and starches; in addition cereal saves the body fat.

- **Caffeine**– has an effect on blood pressure, which could cause problems if you have high blood pressure; in addition, caffeine may make you hungry later. Do not attempt to go "cold turkey" off caffeine as this may cause headaches. Slowly mix in or replace caffeine items with non-caffeine items. If you are a coffee drinker, try to drink it black with Equal® or Splenda®, using no creamer, not even non-dairy creamer.

- **Regular sodas**– many contain caffeine and are high in calories and sugar, which may make you hungry later.

- **Prepackaged frozen meals**– high in calories and most contain items that are not on the *Weight Loss Program*, especially starches and sauces.

- **Protein/energy bars**– high in calories, sugar, and sodium.

- **Pickles**– may be high in sodium.

- **Meal replacement drinks/bars**–high in calories and sodium and many contain items not on the *Weight Loss Program* including soy, dry milk, and corn starch.

- **Alcohol**– high in calories. The average bottle of beer is 150 calories, the average glass of wine is 100 calories, and the average shot of liquor is 120 calories. In addition, the body, sensing alcohol as a form of poison, generates fluid to dilute and remove this poison. Fluid retention causes weight gain and you do not want to do anything that will cause the scale to go up while you are on the *Weight Loss Program*.

Do Not Eat (cont.)

◆ **Pretzels and crackers**– may be high in calories and sodium.

◆ **Canned fruit**– high in calories and sugar.

◆ **Wings (turkey or chicken)**– too fatty.

◆ **Soy**– high in starch. Many people around the world eat soy foods. People in this country are starting to eat them as well. These foods are a good substitute for fatty meats because they contain vegetable protein. They are also low in fat and do not have any cholesterol content.

  The Food and Drug Administration says that a daily diet containing at least 25 grams of soy protein may lower the risk of heart disease. Diets that are high in soy may lower the "bad" cholesterol. The FDA allows foods that contain soy protein to be advertised with the health claim that they reduce the risk of heart disease.

  There has been a concern about soy and an increase in breast cancer. Also a long-term consumption of tofu has been linked to decreased cognitive function and increased brain atrophy in older persons. The risks of allergy are always present and it is thought that soy based infant formulas are not as safe as milk-based formulas.

  However, soy products will not help you lose weight, so do not eat soy products until you are on the *Maintenance Program*.

◆ **Veggie burgers**– most are made with items not on the *Weight Loss Program* including rice, sugar, corn, soy, and oats.

◆ **Catfish**– this is a very fatty fish.

◆ **Popcorn**–corn is one of the starchiest vegetables.

Do Not Eat (cont.)

Some of the Most Fattening Foods:
◆ Peanut butter
◆ Ice cream
◆ Nuts
◆ Glazed donuts
◆ Liver

Supplements

When you are following your *Weight Loss Program*, and eating your meats, vegetables, and fruits, you are essentially providing your body with the necessary vitamins and minerals. However, I do recommend a multivitamin taken with dinner.

Talk to your primary physician about the necessity of adding the following vitamin and mineral supplements to your *Weight Loss Program*.

Vitamins

◆ **Vitamin B12–** important for the normal formation of red blood cells and for the health of the nerve tissues; involved in protein, fat, and carbohydrate metabolism.

Vitamin B12 has been found to make a dieter feel better and have more energy while on a weight loss program. This vitamin is found in the natural form in food and in the synthetic or man-made form in pills and injections. The chemical formulations of the natural and the synthetic vitamin B12 are not the same. The synthetic form is called cyanocobalamin and has a cobalt molecule in its chemical structure. The size of this molecule causes it to be poorly absorbed in the intestine.

In other words, vitamin B12 pills do not work because very little is actually absorbed into the bloodstream. In order to get sufficient vitamin B12 into the bloodstream to make a difference, it must be given by injection. Ask your physician to consent to giving you a vitamin B12 injection in a dose of 500 mcg per week.

◆ **Vitamin C–** a water-soluble vitamin; important in forming collagen, a protein that gives structure to bones, cartilage, muscle, and blood vessels. Vitamin C also helps maintain capillaries, bones, and teeth, heals wounds and burns, helps with bleeding gums, speeds up recovery after surgery, lowers cholesterol, builds the immune system, protects against viral and bacteria infections, extends life, acts as a natural laxative, fights against cancer-causing agents and blood clots, helps with allergies, and aids in the absorption of iron.

◆ **Vitamin E–** a fat-soluble vitamin that protects vitamin A and essential fatty acids from oxidation in the body's cells, prevents breakdown of body tissues, works with vitamin A to help protect lungs against pollution, gives the body oxygen, increases endurance, prevents and dissolves blood clots, helps with fatigue, heals burns, lowers blood pressure, helps to prevent miscarriages, helps with leg cramps, helps fight against heart disease, and prevents thick scarring. Vitamin E also helps to stimulate healthy hair and nail growth.

Minerals

◆ **Calcium–** the most abundant mineral in the body; helps build strong bones and teeth, and is necessary for muscle and nerve functions. Calcium has also been shown to help prevent osteoporosis and help with insomnia.

◆ **Chromium–** the "fat burning pill"; a mineral that has been shown in animal experiments to play an important role in fat metabolism. The implication is that humans who receive an adequate supply of chromium will burn fat faster. The question is, what *is* an adequate supply? It was thought that only a trace of chromium is needed and, therefore, everyone gets enough in their diet. Now researchers are thinking that overweight people do not get enough of this mineral in their diet or that they do not absorb sufficient amounts from their food. There is no proof that chromium capsules increase the rate at which the body burns fat, but it seems to help.

Chromium may also help take the edge off sweet and starch cravings.

Never exceed 400 mcg of chromium in a 24-hour period.

♦ **Iron**– a mineral that is necessary to manufacture hemoglobin which carries oxygen in the blood to the tissues and carbon dioxide back to the lungs for expulsion. Iron aids in growth, promotes resistance to disease, prevents fatigue, cures and prevents iron deficiency anemia, and promotes good skin tone. Iron pills may make you hungry, so if your physician tells you to take iron, take it at night.

♦ **Potassium**– a mineral that helps control acid-base balance in the body, promotes clarity, sends oxygen to the brain, helps to reduce blood pressure, aids in treatment for allergies, works with sodium to regulate water balance, and is used in muscle contraction.

Weight loss involves the loss of some fluid. This is unavoidable and even desirable. However, the loss of fluid often leads to the loss of necessary body potassium. Muscle cramps, cardiac arrest, and death can result if the body potassium level gets too low.

Ask your physician to prescribe an effervescent potassium supplement in the dose of 25 mEq per day. Over-the-counter potassium supplements can be ineffective or dangerous.

Warning About Herbs

Many people think that herbal products are safer than synthetic or man-made medications because herbs come from plants. But we know that some plants are poisonous. Several deaths have been reported due to the use of ephedra (ma huang) and kava, both of which are herbs.

Although herbal products are advertised as "natural," they are not natural to the human body. Unlike prescription medicine, herbal products do not have to be tested to prove that they are safe and effective before they are sold.

In addition, herbal products may not be pure. They may have other ingredients contaminating them, and they may vary from lot to lot. Every 5mg Valium tablet is the same, but every 50mg St. John's Wort capsule may not be the same. You never know.

Herbal medications can also change the way other medicines work and the combination may be even more dangerous than either product is alone. Certain herbs are very dangerous with alcohol.

Here is a short list of some of the more popular herbal products and the side effects that they are proven to cause.

- ◆ **Black cohosh**—Supposed benefit is to help menopausal symptoms such as hot flashes and night sweats. Side effects include headaches, dizziness, nausea, and vision disturbances. The worst effects are in those women who have undiscovered or undiagnosed breast cancer. Black cohosh will worsen breast cancer. If you are not sure whether or not you are suited for synthetic hormone replacement, do not take black cohosh. It can be deadly.

- ◆ **Ephedra (ma huang)**—Supposed benefit is as an energy booster, general stimulant, and appetite suppressant. Proven side effects are hypertension, insomnia, irregular heartbeat, nervousness, tremor, headache, seizure, stroke, kidney stones, heart attack, and death. Ephedra is very dangerous and should never be taken.

◆ **Ginkgo biloba** –Supposed benefit is increased memory. Proven side effect is internal bleeding, especially in patients taking aspirin, aspirin-containing products such as Anacin, and coumadin as a blood thinner. It should not be used.

◆ **Kava**–Supposed benefit is as a sleep aid. Proven side effects are excessive sedation, malfunction of the mouth and tongue, stiff neck, irregular and involuntary movement of the eyes, worsening of the symptoms of Parkinson's disease, and death. It should not be used.

◆ **Senna and licorice root**–Supposed benefit is as a laxative. Proven side effects are lowering of the blood potassium which can lead to irregular heartbeats. It should be used no more than once a month, but only if you are constipated with hard stools.

◆ **St. John's Wort**–Supposed benefit is as an anti-depressant. Proven side effects are gastrointestinal disturbances, allergic reactions, fatigue, dizziness, confusion, dry mouth, and excessive sensitivity to light. Use with care.

Do *not* take any herbal product without first checking with your medical doctor.

WEIGHT LOSS PROGRAM A

Follow Weight Loss Program A every day if you weigh over 230 pounds.

Follow *Weight Loss Program A* and you will lose weight. If you eat or drink something that is not on the program, your weight loss will slow down. Some foods and drinks not on the Allowed Foods may make you hungry, some may make your body store fat instead of burn fat, some may make you retain fluid, and some may make your body manufacture new fat. All of these slow weight loss. Do not skip meals, as that may lead to bingeing.

Following the *Weight Loss Program* is a challenge. It is difficult to stop eating and drinking the things that you like. But "eating to lose" is not how you will have to eat for the rest of your life. You will reach your goal of a healthy weight, you will follow the *Maintenance Program*, you will not have to diet everyday and you will maintain a healthy weight for the rest of your life.

Weight Loss Program A - Instructions

◆ Eat as much as you want from the Allowed Foods list at any-time of the day or night. There are no serving size or quantity restrictions. At your present weight, it is not safe for you to eat a small amount of food. The types of food you eat are more important than the amounts of food you eat.

   If you are allergic to any of the Allowed Foods, do not eat them. You may not, however, substitute them with another food. The meals may be boring, but anything not on your Allowed Foods list will not help you lose weight.

◆ Eat and drink *only* the Allowed Foods. In other words, if something is not on the Allowed Foods list, do not have it, regardless of how "healthy" or "good for you" it is considered. Anything not on your Allowed Foods list will not help you lose weight.

- You *must* eat at least two full meals per day–lunch and dinner. The times of your meals do not matter.
  - A full meal contains Meats, Vegetables, and Fruits selected from the Allowed Foods.
  - Eating just one meal per day will not work.
  - Eating one meal and a salad (just greens) will not work.

- Breakfast– you may have anything from the Allowed Foods. This may take some getting used to as there are no traditional breakfast foods on the list.

- Water– you *must* drink two to three quarts of water per day.

- Snacks – if you get hungry at any time, you may always eat anything on the Allowed Foods list. When you are hungry, even if it is between meals or after dinner, you should eat. Do not starve yourself.

Weight Loss Program A - Allowed Foods

MEATS (may be fresh, canned, or frozen)
There are no serving size or quantity restrictions.

- Chicken breast
- Fish (except for catfish)
- Sardines
- Turkey breast
- Veal
- Crab
- Lobster
- Tuna packed in water
- Shrimp

VEGETABLES (may be fresh, canned, or frozen)
There are no serving size or quantity restrictions.

- Asparagus
- Broccoli
- Cabbage
- Cauliflower
- Collards
- Green peppers
- Lettuce
- Onions
- Spinach
- String beans
- Turnip greens
- Beets
- Brussel sprouts
- Carrots
- Celery
- Cucumbers
- Kale
- Mushrooms
- Peas
- Squash
- Tomatoes
- Zucchini

Note: Do not use canned vegetables flavored with extra sodium, pork, or other meat products.

FRUITS (must be fresh, *no* canned or frozen fruit)
There are no serving size or quantity restrictions.

- Apples
- Cantaloupes
- Grapes
- Oranges
- Pears
- Strawberries
- Bananas
- Grapefruits
- Nectarines
- Peaches
- Prunes
- Tangerines

DRINKS

There are no serving size or quantity restrictions.

- Water
- Sugar free, caffeine free diet sodas
- Herb teas
- Decaffeinated coffee

Weight Loss Program A – Exercise

While you are on *Weight Loss Program A*, you do not have to follow a strict exercise regimen. At your present weight, the walking involved in your day-to-day activities is enough exercise. Walking outside, around the mall, or on the treadmill with no incline for a maximum of 15 minutes, 3 days a week is okay, but not necessary. Water aerobics, stretching, yoga, and pilates at the beginner's level are also okay.

It could be dangerous and damaging to your knees, back, hips, and heart if you engage in vigorous exercise such as running, lifting weights, high impact aerobics, stair climbing, and riding a bicycle.

Weight Loss Program A - If You Get Hungry

While you are on *Weight Loss Program A*, if you get hungry–eat! Just make sure it is something on your Allowed Foods list. Do not skip lunch and do not skip dinner. Always have meats, vegetables, and fruits with each meal. Plan ahead for your meals and plan ahead for your snacks. Have something from your Allowed Foods for breakfast.

At this time you do not have to fight or deal with being hungry. If you get hungry in between meals or if you get hungry after dinner or if you get hungry in the middle of the night, always eat something on your Allowed Foods list. Do not starve yourself.

Weight Loss Program A - If You Reach a Plateau

You have reached a plateau when you lose less than 8 pounds per month or your weight has remained the same for 3 weeks. Follow these steps in order to break out of a plateau. Once you begin to lose weight again, you may stop following the steps for a plateau. In other words, if you implement Step 2 and your weight loss resumes, then you do not have to continue onto Step 3.

Step 1 - Review the Allowed Foods list. Sometimes after being on a diet, you tend to forget which foods are allowed and which foods are not allowed.

Follow *Weight Loss Program A* exactly for 7 out of 7 days. Not 5 or even 6 out of 7 days, but every meal of every day.

Review the introduction to this book, *The Diet Salon*.

Step 2 - Keep a *Food Diary* for a week. See a sample *Food Diary* in Appendix C. Compare your *Food Diary* with your Allowed Foods to verify that you are not eating something that is not on your Allowed Foods list.

Verify that you are eating lunch and dinner, and not skipping meals. Skipping meals leads to low blood sugar causing hunger pains that may lead to bingeing and the craving for "heavy food." This will not help you lose weight.

Verify that you are eating the meats, vegetables, and fruits for each meal.

Verify that you are drinking two to three quarts of water per day.

Step 3 - Your present weight may be on the cusp of *Weight Loss Program A*. Switch to *Weight Loss Program B*. For example, if your weight plateaus at 235 pounds, then it is time to switch to *Weight Loss Program B*.

Step 4 - Consult a bariatric physician–a licensed physician who offers specialized programs in the medical treatment of obesity and its associated conditions. This type of physician can give you appetite suppressants and vitamin B12 injections to help you stay on the diet.

In D.C., Baltimore, and Richmond contact:

Robert S. Beale, Jr., M.D.
1712 I Street, NW
Suite 604
Washington, DC 20006
Phone: 202-463-7872
Website: www.docbeale.com

In Atlanta and Albany, Georgia contact:

J. Tom Cooper, M.D.
1234 Powers Ferry Road
Suite 104
Marietta, GA 30067
Phone (Atlanta): 770-952-7681
Phone (Albany): 229-439-0904

In Detroit, Michigan contact:

Bill Nagler, M.D.
16311 Middlebelt Road
Livonia, MI 48154
Phone: 734-422-8040

In New York, New York contact:

Gary Zisk, D.O.
8223 Bay Parkway
Brooklyn, NY 11214
Phone: 718-259-1979

For physicians in other areas contact the American Society of Bariatric Physicians on the Web at www.asbp.org or by phone at 303-770-2526.

Step 5 - If no bariatric physician is located in your area, consult your primary care physician.

WEIGHT LOSS PROGRAM B

Follow Weight Loss Program B every day if you weigh from 191 pounds to 230 pounds.

Follow *Weight Loss Program B* and you will lose weight. If you eat or drink something that is not on the program, your weight loss will slow down. Some foods and drinks not on the Allowed Foods may make you hungry, some may make your body store fat instead of burn fat, some may make you retain fluid, and some may make your body manufacture new fat. All of these slow weight loss. Do not skip meals, as that may lead to bingeing.

Following the *Weight Loss Program* is a challenge. It is difficult to stop eating and drinking the things that you like. But "eating to lose" is not how you will have to eat for the rest of your life. You will reach your goal of a healthy weight, you will follow the *Maintenance Program*, you will not have to diet everyday and you will maintain a healthy weight for the rest of your life.

Weight Loss Program B - Instructions

◆ Eat as much as you want from the Allowed Foods list at anytime of the day or night. There are no serving size or quantity restrictions. At your present weight, it is not safe for you to eat a small amount of food. The types of food you eat are more important than the amount of food you eat.

   If you are allergic to any of the Allowed Foods, do not eat them. You may not, however, substitute them with another food. The meals may be boring, but anything not on your Allowed Foods list will not help you lose weight.

◆ Eat and drink *only* the Allowed Foods. In other words, if something is not on the Allowed Foods list, do not have it, regardless of how "healthy" or "good for you" it is considered. Anything not on the Allowed Foods list will not help you lose weight.

◆ You *must* eat at least two full meals per day–lunch and dinner. The times of your meals do not matter.

  ◆ A full meal contains Meats, Vegetables, and Fruits selected from the Allowed Foods.

  ◆ Eating just one meal per day will not work.

  ◆ Eating one meal and a salad (just greens) will not work.

◆ Breakfast– you may have anything from the Allowed Foods. This may take some getting used to as there are no traditional breakfast foods on the list.

◆ Water– you *must* drink two to three quarts of water per day.

◆ Snacks– if you get hungry at anytime, you may always eat anything on the Allowed Foods list. When you are hungry, even if it is between meals or after dinner, you should eat. Do not starve yourself.

Weight Loss Program B - Allowed Foods

MEATS (may be fresh, canned, or frozen)
There are no serving size or quantity restrictions.

◆ Chicken breast
◆ Fish (except for catfish)
◆ Tuna packed in water
◆ Shrimp

◆ Crab
◆ Lobster
◆ Turkey breast

VEGETABLES (may be fresh, canned, or frozen)
There are no serving size or quantity restrictions.

- Asparagus
- Brussel sprouts
- Celery
- Cucumbers
- Kale
- Onions
- Turnip greens
- Broccoli
- Cabbage
- Collards
- Green peppers
- Lettuce
- Spinach

Note: Do not use canned vegetables flavored with extra sodium, pork, or other meat products.

FRUITS (must be fresh, *no* canned or frozen fruit)
There are no serving size or quantity restrictions.

- Apples
- Grapes
- Strawberries
- Grapefruits
- Oranges

DRINKS
There are no serving size or quantity restrictions.

- Water
- Sugar free, caffeine free diet sodas
- Herb teas
- Decaffeinated coffee

Weight Loss Program B – Exercise

While you are on *Weight Loss Program B*, you do not have to follow a strict exercise regimen. At your present weight, the walking involved in your day-to-day activities is enough exercise. Walking outside, around the mall, or on the treadmill with no incline for a maximum of 15 minutes, 3 days a week is okay, but not necessary. Water aerobics, stretching, yoga, and pilates at the beginner's level are also okay.

It could be dangerous and damaging to your knees, back, hips, and heart if you engage in vigorous exercise such as running, lifting weights, high impact aerobics, stair climbing, and riding a bicycle.

Weight Loss Program B - If You Get Hungry

While you are on *Weight Loss Program B*, if you get hungry–eat! Just make sure it is something on your Allowed Foods list. Do not skip lunch and do not skip dinner. Always have meats, vegetables, and fruits with each meal. Plan ahead for your meals and plan ahead for your snacks. Have something from your Allowed Foods for breakfast.

At this time you do not have to fight or deal with being hungry. If you get hungry in between meals or if you get hungry after dinner or if you get hungry in the middle of the night, always eat something on your Allowed Foods list. Do not starve yourself.

Weight Loss Program B - If You Reach a Plateau

You have reached a plateau when you lose less than 8 pounds per month or your weight has remained the same for 3 weeks. Follow these steps in order to break out of a plateau. Once you begin to lose weight again, you may stop following the steps for a plateau. In other words, if you implement Step 2 and your weight loss resumes, then you do not have to continue onto Step 3.

Step 1 - Review the Allowed Foods list. Sometimes after being on a diet, you tend to forget which foods are allowed and which foods are not allowed.

Follow *Weight Loss Program B* exactly for 7 out of 7 days. Not 5 or even 6 out of 7 days, but every meal of every day.

Review the introduction to this book, *The Diet Salon*.

Step 2 - Keep a *Food Diary* for a week. See a sample *Food Diary* in Appendix C. Compare your *Food Diary* with your Allowed Foods to verify that you are not eating something that is not on your Allowed Foods list.

Verify that you are eating lunch and dinner, and not skipping meals. Skipping meals leads to low blood sugar causing hunger pains that may lead to bingeing and the craving for "heavy food." This will not help you lose weight.

Verify that you are eating the meats, vegetables, and fruits for each meal.

Verify that you are drinking two to three quarts of water per day.

Step 3 - Your present weight may be on the cusp of *Weight Loss Program B*. Switch to *Weight Loss Program C*. For example, if your weight plateaus at 195 pounds, then it is time to switch to *Weight Loss Program C*.

Step 4 - Consult a bariatric physician–a licensed physician who offers specialized programs in the medical treatment of obesity and its associated conditions. This type of physician can give you appetite suppressants and vitamin B12 injections to help you stay on the diet.

In D.C., Baltimore, and Richmond contact:

Robert S. Beale, Jr., M.D.
1712 I Street, NW
Suite 604
Washington, DC 20006
Phone: 202-463-7872
Website: www.docbeale.com

In Atlanta and Albany, Georgia contact:

J. Tom Cooper, M.D.
1234 Powers Ferry Road
Suite 104
Marietta, GA 30067
Phone (Atlanta): 770-952-7681
Phone (Albany): 229-439-0904

In Detroit, Michigan contact:

Bill Nagler, M.D.
16311 Middlebelt Road
Livonia, MI 48154
Phone: 734-422-8040

In New York, New York contact:

Gary Zisk, D.O.
8223 Bay Parkway
Brooklyn, NY 11214
Phone: 718-259-1979

For physicians in other areas contact the American Society of Bariatric Physicians on the Web at www.asbp.org or by phone at 303-770-2526.

Step 5 - If no bariatric physician is located in your area, consult your primary care physician.

WEIGHT LOSS PROGRAM C

Follow Weight Loss Program C every day if you weigh from 160 pounds to 190 pounds.

Follow *Weight Loss Program C* and you will lose weight. If you eat or drink something that is not on the program, your weight loss will slow down. Some foods and drinks not on the Allowed Foods may make you hungry, some may make your body store fat instead of burn fat, some may make you retain fluid, and some may make your body manufacture new fat. All of these slow weight loss. Do not skip meals, as that may lead to bingeing.

Following the *Weight Loss Program* is a challenge. It is difficult to stop eating and drinking the things that you like. But "eating to lose" is not how you will have to eat for the rest of your life. You will reach your goal of a healthy weight, you will follow the *Maintenance Program*, you will not have to diet everyday and you will maintain a healthy weight for the rest of your life.

Weight Loss Program C - Instructions

◆ Eat and drink *only* those items on the Allowed Foods list. Consume no more than the specified serving sizes. If something is not on the Allowed Foods list, do not have it regardless of how "healthy" or "good for you" it is considered. Anything not on the Allowed Foods list will not help lose weight.

If you are allergic to any of the Allowed Foods, do not eat them. You may not, however, substitute them with another food. The meals may be boring, but anything not on your Allowed Foods list will not help you lose weight.

◆ You *must* eat two full meals per day–lunch and dinner. The times of your meals do not matter.
   ◆ A full meal contains Meats, Vegetables, and Fruits selected from the Allowed Foods.
   ◆ Eating just 1 meal per day will not work.
   ◆ Eating 1 meal and a salad (just greens) will not work.

- Water–you ***must*** drink two to three quarts of water per day.

- Breakfast (optional)–you may have only one of the following:
    - 1 serving from the Meats OR
    - 1 serving from the Vegetables OR
    - 1 serving from the Fruits OR
    - You may take three slices of turkey breast, roll them individually around some lettuce, and use a fat-free salad dressing or mustard as dip.

  This may take some getting used to as there are no traditional breakfast foods on the list.

- Snacks (optional)–you may have up to two snacks per day at any time, including until the time you go to bed. You may have only one of the following per snack:
    - 1 serving from the Meats OR
    - 1 serving from the Vegetables OR
    - 1 serving from the Fruits OR
    - You may take three slices of turkey breast, roll them individually around lettuce, and use a fat-free salad dressing or mustard as dip.

Weight Loss Program C - Allowed Foods

MEATS (may be fresh, canned, or frozen)
Each serving is 6 – 8 ounces.

- Chicken breast
- Fish (except for catfish)
- Tuna packed in water
- Shrimp
- Crab
- Lobster
- Turkey breast

VEGETABLES (may be fresh, canned, or frozen)
Each serving is 1.5 – 2 cups. You may combine different vegetables as long as the total volume is within 2 cups.

- Asparagus
- Cabbage
- Collards
- Green peppers
- Lettuce
- Spinach

- Broccoli
- Celery
- Cucumbers
- Kale
- Onions
- Turnip greens

Note: Do not use canned vegetables flavored with extra sodium, pork, or other meat products.

FRUITS (must be fresh, *no* canned or frozen fruit)

- Apples–1 large
- Grapes–up to 18
- Strawberries–up to 10

- Grapefruits–1 large
- Oranges–1 large

DRINKS
There are no serving size or quantity restrictions.

- Water
- Sugar free, caffeine free diet sodas
- Herb teas
- Decaffeinated coffee

Weight Loss Program C – Exercise
While you are on *Weight Loss Program C*, you do not have to follow a strict exercise regimen as long as you are losing weight. Walking outside, around the mall, or on the treadmill with no incline for 30 minutes, 3 times a week is okay. Water aerobics, elliptical machines, stretching, yoga, and pilates at the beginner's level are also okay.

Engaging in vigorous exercise such as running, lifting weights, stair climbing, high impact aerobics, or riding a bicycle maybe too much for your body's frame to handle, and it will build too much muscle. You may notice that you are getting firm, but that you are also getting bulky. You may also notice that the scale is not going down. Walking is the best exercise to help you tone without putting too much stress on your frame and without building too much muscle.

Weight Loss Program C - If You Get Hungry

While you are on *Weight Loss Program C*, make sure that you are not skipping lunch and that you are not skipping dinner. Always have meats, vegetables, and fruits with each meal. Have something from your Allowed Foods for breakfast and eat both of your snacks. Plan ahead for your meals and plan ahead for your snacks.

Weight Loss Program C - If You Reach a Plateau

You have reached a plateau when you lose less than 8 pounds per month or your weight has remained the same for 3 weeks. Follow these steps in order to break out of a plateau. Once you begin to lose weight again, you may stop following the steps for a plateau. In other words, if you implement Step 2 and your weight loss resumes, then you do not have to continue onto Step 3.

Step 1 - Review the Allowed Foods list. Sometimes after being on a diet, you tend to forget which foods are allowed and which foods are not allowed.

Follow *Weight Loss Program C* exactly for 7 out of 7 days. Not 5 or even 6 out of 7 days, but every meal of every day.

Review the introduction to this book, *The Diet Salon*.

Step 2 - Keep a *Food Diary* for a week. See a sample *Food Diary* in Appendix C. Compare your *Food Diary* with your Allowed Foods to verify that you are not eating something that is not on your Allowed Foods list.

Verify that you are eating lunch and dinner, and not skipping meals. Skipping meals leads to low blood sugar causing hunger pains that may lead to bingeing and the craving for "heavy food." This will not help you lose weight.

Verify that you are eating the meats, vegetables, and fruits for each meal.

Verify that you are drinking two to three quarts of water per day.

Step 3 - Reduce the number of snacks to 1 versus 2 per day.

Step 4 - Your present weight may be on the cusp of *Weight Loss Program C*. Switch to *Weight Loss Program D*. For example, if your weight plateaus at 165 pounds, then it is time to switch to *Weight Loss Program D*.

Step 5 - Consult a bariatric physician–a licensed physician who offers specialized programs in the medical treatment of obesity and its associated conditions. This type of physician can give you appetite suppressants and vitamin B12 injections to help you stay on the diet.

In D.C., Baltimore, and Richmond contact:

Robert S. Beale, Jr., M.D.
1712 I Street, NW
Suite 604
Washington, DC 20006
Phone: 202-463-7872
Website: www.docbeale.com

In Atlanta and Albany, Georgia contact:

J. Tom Cooper, M.D.
1234 Powers Ferry Road
Suite 104
Marietta, GA 30067
Phone (Atlanta): 770-952-7681
Phone (Albany): 229-439-0904

In Detroit, Michigan contact:

Bill Nagler, M.D.
16311 Middlebelt Road
Livonia, MI 48154
Phone: 734-422-8040

In New York, New York contact:

Gary Zisk, D.O.
8223 Bay Parkway
Brooklyn, NY 11214
Phone: 718-259-1979

For physicians in other areas contact the American Society of Bariatric Physicians on the Web at www.asbp.org or by phone at 303-770-2526.

Step 6 - If no bariatric physician is located in your area, consult your primary care physician.

WEIGHT LOSS PROGRAM D

Follow Weight Loss Program D every day if you weigh less than 160 pounds.

Follow *Weight Loss Program D* and you will lose weight. If you eat or drink something that is not on the program, your weight loss will slow down. Some foods and drinks not on the Allowed Foods may make you hungry, some may make your body store fat instead of burn fat, some may make you retain fluid, and some may make your body manufacture new fat. All of these slow weight loss. Do not skip meals, as that may lead to bingeing.

Following the *Weight Loss Program* is a challenge. It is difficult to stop eating and drinking the things that you like. But "eating to lose" is not how you will have to eat for the rest of your life. You will reach your goal of a healthy weight, you will follow the *Maintenance Program*, you will not have to diet everyday and you will maintain a healthy weight for the rest of your life.

Weight Loss Program D - Instructions

◆ Eat and drink *only* those items on the Allowed Foods list. Consume no more than the specified serving sizes. If something is not on the Allowed Foods list, do not have it regardless of how "healthy" or "good for you" it is considered. Anything not on the Allowed Foods list will not help lose weight.

If you are allergic to any of the Allowed Foods, do not eat them. You may not, however, substitute them with another food. The meals may be boring, but anything not on your Allowed Foods list will not help you lose weight.

◆ You *must* eat two full meals per day – lunch and dinner. The times of your meals do not matter.
  ◆ A full meal contains Meats, Vegetables, and Fruits selected from the Allowed Foods.
  ◆ Eating just 1 meal per day will not work.
  ◆ Eating 1 meal and a salad (just greens) will not work.

◆ Water–you *must* drink two to three quarts of water per day.

◆ Breakfast (optional)–you may have only 1 of the following:
   ◆ 1 serving from the Meats OR
   ◆ 1 serving from the Vegetables OR
   ◆ 1 serving from the Fruits OR
   ◆ You may take two slices of turkey breast, roll them individually around lettuce, and use a fat-free salad dressing or mustard as dip.

This may take some getting used to as there are no traditional breakfast foods on the list.

◆ Snacks (optional)–you may have only one snack per day at any time, including until the time you go to bed. You may have only one of the following per snack:
   ◆ 1 serving from the Meats OR
   ◆ 1 serving from the Vegetables OR
   ◆ 1 serving from the Fruits OR
   ◆ You may take two slices of turkey breast, roll them individually around lettuce, and use a fat-free salad dressing or mustard as dip.

Weight Loss Program D - Allowed Foods

MEATS (may be fresh, canned, or frozen)
Each serving is 4 – 6 ounces.

◆ Chicken breast
◆ Fish (except for catfish)
◆ Tuna packed in water
◆ Shrimp
◆ Crab
◆ Lobster
◆ Turkey breast

VEGETABLES (may be fresh, canned, or frozen)
Each serving is 1 – 1.5 cups. You may combine different vegetables as long as the total volume is within 1.5 cups.

- Asparagus
- Cabbage
- Collards
- Green peppers
- Lettuce
- Spinach

- Broccoli
- Celery
- Cucumbers
- Kale
- Onions
- Turnip greens

Note: Do not use canned vegetables flavored with extra sodium, pork, or other meat products.

FRUITS (must be fresh, *no* canned or frozen fruit)

- Apples – 1 large
- Grapes – up to 12
- Strawberries – up to 8

- Grapefruits – $1/2$ of a large
- Oranges – 1 large

DRINKS

There are no serving size or quantity restrictions.

- Water
- Sugar free, caffeine free diet sodas
- Herb teas
- Decaffeinated coffee

Weight Loss Program D – Exercise

While you are on *Weight Loss Program D*, you do not have to follow a strict exercise regimen as long as you are losing weight. Walking outside, around the mall, or on the treadmill with no incline for 30 – 45 minutes every other day is okay. Water aerobics, elliptical machines, stretching, yoga, and pilates are okay.

As you get close to your goal weight, you must make a decision as to how you want your body to look. Do you want to be lean and toned or do you want to look like a professional athlete? Do you want to look better in your clothes or out of your clothes?

Engaging in vigorous exercise such as running, lifting weights, stair climbing, high impact aerobics, or riding a bicycle will build muscle and can cause damage to your body's frame if you have not been properly trained. Be very aware of how your body changes if you do these exercises. Make sure you are getting the results you want.

You may notice that you are getting firm, but that you are also getting bulky. You may also notice that the scale is not going down. Walking and using very light weights are the best exercises to help you tone without building too much muscle.

Weight Loss Program D - If You Get Hungry

While you are on *Weight Loss Program D*, make sure that you are not skipping lunch and that you are not skipping dinner. Always have the proper serving size of meats, vegetables, and fruits with each meal. Have something from your Allowed Foods for breakfast and eat your one snack. Plan ahead for your meals and plan ahead for your snack.

You will not be on *Weight Loss Program D* for long, really no more than a few months. Following *Weight Loss Program D* is challenging, but with proper planning, you will reach your goal in the short term.

For runners only: If you run more than two miles at least three times a week, you may add a small saucer of plain pasta with no sauce the night before the days that you run.

Weight Loss Program D - If You Reach a Plateau

You have reached a plateau when you lose less than 5 pounds per month or your weight has remained the same for 3 weeks. Follow these steps in order to break out of a plateau. Once you begin to lose weight again, you may stop following the steps for a plateau. In other words, if you implement Step 2 and your weight loss resumes, then you do not have to continue onto Step 3.

Step 1 - Review the Allowed Foods list. Sometimes after being on a diet, you tend to forget which foods are allowed and which foods are not allowed.

Follow *Weight Loss Program D* exactly for 7 out of 7 days. Not 5 or even 6 out of 7 days, but every meal of every day.

Review the introduction to this book, *The Diet Salon.*

Step 2 - Keep a *Food Diary* for a week. See a sample *Food Diary* in Appendix C. Compare your *Food Diary* with your Allowed Foods to verify that you are not eating something that is not on your Allowed Foods list.

Verify that you are eating the meats, vegetables, and fruits for each meal.

Verify that you are drinking two to three quarts of water per day.

Verify that you are eating enough and not skipping meals. Skipping meals leads to low blood sugar causing hunger pains that may lead to bingeing and the craving for "heavy food." This will not help you lose weight.

Step 3 - Change your serving sizes to the following:

* Meat – 4 ounces
* Vegetables – 1 cup
* Fruits – 1 medium apple, 1 medium orange, 1/2 grapefruit, 10 grapes, 6 strawberries

Step 4 - Do not have a snack for a few days.

Step 5 - Increase your level of activity. If you are not walking on a regular basis, start walking for 30 minutes 3 times a week. If you are already walking for exercise, increase the time you walk by 10 to 15 minutes and increase the frequency as your schedule allows.

Step 6 - If you have reached a healthy weight but you are within 5–10 pounds of your goal, reconsider your goal. It is definitely possible to reach your goal, but sometimes it is not worth the sacrifice to be that small. You have to decide for yourself.

You may go on the *Maintenance Program* for a while, so that you will not have to diet every day for the time being. When you have maintained your modified goal weight for a few months, if you decide that you still want to lose those last few pounds, then start following *Weight Loss Program D* again. It should take no more than six weeks to reach your original goal.

Step 7 - Consult a bariatric physician–a licensed physician who offers specialized programs in the medical treatment of obesity and its associated conditions. This type of physician can give you appetite suppressants and vitamin B12 injections to help you stay on the diet.

In D.C., Baltimore, and Richmond contact:

Robert S. Beale, Jr., M.D.
1712 I Street, NW
Suite 604
Washington, DC 20006
Phone: 202-463-7872
Website: www.docbeale.com

In Atlanta and Albany, Georgia contact:

J. Tom Cooper, M.D.
1234 Powers Ferry Road
Suite 104
Marietta, GA 30067
Phone (Atlanta): 770-952-7681
Phone (Albany): 229-439-0904

In Detroit, Michigan contact:

Bill Nagler, M.D.
16311 Middlebelt Road
Livonia, MI 48154
Phone: 734-422-8040

In New York, New York contact:

Gary Zisk, D.O.
8223 Bay Parkway
Brooklyn, NY 11214
Phone: 718-259-1979

For physicians in other areas contact the American Society of Bariatric Physicians on the Web at www.asbp.org or by phone at 303-770-2526.

Step 8 - If no bariatric physician is located in your area, consult your primary care physician.

Four

Weight Loss Strategies

This information is helpful for continued weight loss, whether you are on *Weight Loss Program A, Weight Loss Program B, Weight Loss Program C,* or *Weight Loss Program D.*

You Are Not a Dieting Machine

Life does not stop because you are on a diet. You are not the perfect dieting machine. There are still stressful times, business functions, birthday parties, holidays, and vacations. As with life, some days are better than others and some weeks are better than others. Do the best you can. If you go off your *Weight Loss Program* for a day or even a few days, do not beat yourself up, do not panic, and try not to feel guilty. Just get right back on track and you will continue to lose weight.

Almost no one can follow the *Weight Loss Program* for weeks without "cheating." You should treat this as if it were a course in school. If you do not get 100 on each test, that is not a reason to drop the course. You try harder the next time. Unlike a course, however, doing "extra credit" will not improve your progress. Lifting heavy weights or running five miles per day may not help you lose weight, especially if you are not following your *Weight Loss Program.* This vigorous exercise could also be very dangerous.

Getting to your goal weight may take a long time. With every 10 pounds you lose, you will feel better, sleep better, breathe better, get around better and you will generally be healthier. Try to remember how long it sometimes takes when you are at the hair salon, especially if you are getting braids. It is difficult to be sitting in the chair all of that time, but in the end it is all worth it.

The Time of Day to Eat Your Meals

Eat your meals at a time that is convenient for you, the time does not matter. All of the *Weight Loss Programs* require a minimum of 2 full meals with meat, vegetables, and fruit per day. This means that you must eat lunch and dinner. Your meal times will vary depending on your family, work, church, or school schedule. For example, if you work at night, that may mean having "lunch" at 1 a.m. and "dinner" at 7 a.m. If you are in class until 9 p.m., that may mean having a snack before you go to class, and then eating dinner later.

If you get home late and you have not had dinner, still eat dinner. Now you would not want to eat spaghetti and meatballs before going to bed, but luckily those foods are not on the *Weight Loss Program*. It is better to eat dinner with the foods on your *Weight Loss Program* than to not eat at all.

When you skip a meal, it sends your body into starvation mode. As a defense mechanism, the body slows down your metabolism and starts storing food. It does not take skipping too many meals before you either go off your diet because you are hungry or you get sick.

Meal Preparation

Figuring out what to eat when you are hungry and have no time to cook is a challenge. For lunch when time is minimal, that means you are left to hopefully find something at the cafeteria, if it is still open, or you must leave the premises to hunt for a meal that contains only the foods on your *Weight Loss Program*. For dinner at the end of a hectic day, that means while driving home you must stop somewhere along the way to pick something up. This can spell trouble in the world of fast food and take out.

Plan Ahead

Having your food available when it is time to eat makes following the *Weight Loss Program* much easier. Go to the grocery store once a week, preferably at the beginning, and buy enough food for breakfast, lunch, dinner, and snacks for the entire week. Prepare some food, such as chopped baked chicken breast or a pot of cabbage, that can be stored and eaten throughout the week. Purchase frozen food, such as grilled frozen fish fillets and frozen vegetables to eat when you have no time or desire to actually cook a meal.

Finding the time to eat lunch–and even figuring out what to eat for lunch–may be difficult. During those busy days, you check your watch and it is already after 2 p.m. A good strategy for lunch is to take it with you. To save even more time in the morning, pack your lunch at night. As a reminder to bring it with you, put your keys on top of your lunch in the refrigerator. (If that means that you will also forget where you put your keys, then leave a note for yourself on your purse.)

Make something for lunch that is easy to eat, something that you can either eat in 10 minutes or eat a few bites at a time over the course of an hour. Try foods that require only a fork to eat such as tuna over lettuce and grapes versus a whole grilled chicken breast and an orange which require a knife for cutting and fingers for peeling. Set an automatic reminder on your system calendar, phone, or handheld device to remind you to eat midday.

Eating dinner is a must, no matter what time you go to sleep. It is better to eat a dinner from the foods on your *Weight Loss Program* and go right to bed than to not eat at all. Always have an easy emergency meal available. Frozen foods and foods that have been prepared ahead of time work best. All that is required when you are tired and hungry is to put the plate in the microwave, no buying groceries or cooking is necessary.

Keeping a Food Diary

Keeping a Food Diary of all the food and drinks you consume each day can be very helpful. This diary should be kept with you at all times. Write down all food and drinks before you eat or drink them. Once you write something down, if you think that you should not consume it, then leave it out and mark through the entry.

Each week when you record your weight, compare your Food Diary with your *Weight Loss Program*. Verify that you are eating your meals with meats, vegetables and fruits from your Allowed Foods, that you are drinking two to three quarts of water per day, and that you are eating only the snacks allowed on your *Weight Loss Program*. You will be able to see how much you lose when you are closer to following your *Weight Loss Program* than when you are not. See Appendix C for a sample *Food Diary*.

Lose Weight with a Friend

If you have a friend who also wants to lose weight, you can go on this journey together, supporting each other along the way.

- Share ideas.

- Encourage each other.

- Talk about challenges and solutions.

- Take turns cooking. Perhaps one day you make enough food for the both of you to have lunch, then the next day it is her turn.

- Take walks.

- Spend time together socially without the pressure of the "diet police" or the "feeder."

- Most of all, be a good listener.

Fasting for Religious Reasons

In both the Christian and Muslim religions, fasting for spiritual reasons is an important ritual that is undertaken for various reasons. Fasting may be done at any time for personal cleansing, as a supplication to God for prayers to be answered, as thanks for prayers answered or deliverance from danger, as a part of a High Holy Season, or for many other reasons.

In the traditional case, the fasting person intakes no food or water for an extended period of time. However, today most religious leaders recognize that the traditional fast can be dangerous for most of their worshippers. Therefore, revised versions are offered. The most common are: abstaining from solid foods but intaking liquids such as soups and juices; avoiding all intake for a short period of time such as from sunup to sundown, but allowing all foods after sundown; or a variation permitting juices but no other liquids or solids for a short period of time such as a few days.

All of these fasting regimens are good for spiritual reasons, but do nothing for weight loss. Soups and juices are a good source of calories and hence save the body fat. That is why these fasts are usually safe for a short period of time. When your religion calls for fasting, you must suspend your attempt to lose weight, but then resume your *Weight Loss Program* once the fasting period is over.

Eating on a Budget

Use canned tuna, frozen grilled fish fillets, and chicken. Buy the chicken whole if you have others in your household. You eat the breast and leave the rest for the others. Use frozen vegetables because they last longer. Use the fruits that are in season: apples and oranges are usually less expensive. Comparison shop, especially if you have access to warehouse food clubs. Look for "weekly specials" in the grocery store circular.

Eating with Your Family

When you are preparing meals for your family, make sure you have a snack available to munch on while you are cooking. Sliced cucumbers work well. Utilize spices so that the food is not so bland. Let family members put the starch portion on their plate in the kitchen instead of placing it on the dining table.

If you cook something for your family that is not on your *Weight Loss Program*, have your meal already prepared. You do not want to have to cook two separate dishes.

Try some of the recipes in *Appendix B*. Many of them are so flavorful that your family may not even realize they are eating "diet food."

Eating at Catered Functions
Eating with Colleagues
Eating at Restaurants

Your colleagues and acquaintances do not need to know that you are on a diet. Order the baked, grilled or blackened fish, steamed vegetables, or grilled chicken salad. Sometimes you will be in a situation where you must eat food that is not on your *Weight Loss Program*. Try to stay away from or eat as little as possible of the starches. If given the choice, do not get dessert unless there is a fruit plate. Drink plenty of water.

For cocktail hour, choose sparkling mineral water on the rocks with a twist or a diet soda instead of alcohol.

These situations need not be awkward; do the best you can with the available options. When you are back in an environment that you can control, get right back on your *Weight Loss Program* and follow it exactly.

Eating at a Dinner Party

Before going to a dinner party, have a snack according to your *Weight Loss Program*. This way you are not quite so hungry when you arrive. When the appetizers are served, pass on all except for the vegetables. Instead of a cocktail, have a sparkling mineral water on the rocks with a twist or a diet soda. Participating more in conversation and mingling with other guests will help you stay clear of the food.

At the table, fill your own plate if possible, getting large portions of vegetables and salad, and small portions of the rest. Avoid the starches, especially the bread. Compliment your hostess or host on the meal as you turn down offers for second helpings. You do not have to overeat to be a gracious guest.

Eating on a Business Trip

When you have the option to eat at your hotel, order room service. Tell the kitchen that you want baked, grilled or blackened fish, steamed vegetables, or grilled chicken salad. Also order the fruit plate, letting them know which fruits to include. Even if these items are not specifically on the menu, most hotels will accommodate your request.

Eating When You Have a 14+ Hour Day Away from Home

When your schedule includes taking your children to school, working all day, going to class at night, or working on a project with a tight deadline, there is not much time to figure out what to eat. You must go to the grocery store before the week starts and stock up on all of your food for the entire week. Prepare foods that you can warm up and eat over several days.

Get items that travel well and do not require refrigeration such as tuna packaged in a bag, apples, celery, and lettuce. Do not forget to prepare and bring your snack with you. Have frozen foods or meals already on a plate available for those times when you get home late at night.

Eating on a Road Trip

When you are traveling by car or by bus on a long road trip, take meals, snacks, and water with you. If possible, when stops are made, avoid getting in the fast food line.

Take Out and Fast Food

Be extremely aware of the contents and preparation of take out and fast food meals. The food in many Asian and southern style take out establishments contains sodium and calorie-filled sauces. It is recommended that you do not eat these items, even if it is chicken and broccoli, due to its preparation.

Make sure that the salad from a take out or fast food establishment contains only those foods on your *Weight Loss Program*. Many times salad dressings are not fat free, so you will have to use your own.

When ordering a grilled chicken breast that comes only in sandwich form, immediately throw the bread away before sitting down to eat.

Drinking Water

You must drink at least two to three quarts of water per day.

Most water drinkers are not born, you have to "become" a water drinker. However, once you become a water drinker, it is not that bad.

- Try drinking a glass of water every hour.

- Use your system calendar, phone, or handheld device to set a reminder. Over the course of the day you will drink two to three quarts.

- Try water at different temperatures. Room temperature water may go down a little easier especially during cold weather.

◆ Try using a cup or a widemouth bottle. Drinking out of a bottle with a small opening may cause you to swallow excess air.

◆ You may also add fresh lemon, but do not make lemonade!

When You Are Bored with the Food or Just Bored in General

The foods on the diet are not very exciting. However, following the *Weight Loss Programs* is "eating to lose." It is not the way you will have to eat forever.

Try different spice blends such as garlic and herb, lemon and pepper, Caribbean Jerk, and Cajun to add variety. Also, cook different types of fish and use your seafood options several times a week.

You may not look forward to meals now as much as before. They become more of a task, like brushing your teeth. When you are finished eating the meal on your *Weight Loss Program*, then you move on to something more exciting.

Engage in new activities in order to help you get through that bored feeling. Here are some suggestions:

◆ Learn a new language

◆ Try a new hobby–arts, crafts, collecting

◆ Call a relative or friend

◆ Take a walk

◆ Spend time with a child

◆ Go to the library

◆ Volunteer

◆ Get a facial, massage, manicure, or pedicure

◆ Learn yoga or pilates

◆ Write a letter

◆ Read a book

When You Wake Up Hungry in the Middle of the Night

If you are prone to haunting the kitchen at midnight in search of food, always have something prepared so that it is immediately available. Either have a small plate with leftovers from dinner, or prepare one of the Snacks from Appendix B - *Recipes*.

Waking up hungry in the middle of the night can be an indication that you may not be eating enough during the day, especially at dinner. Make sure that you eat the reccommended serving sizes of meats, vegetables, and fruits, and your minimum two full meals for your *Weight Loss Program*.

How to Deal with Cravings

Cravings often happen around the time of your period, when you are bored, when you are stressed, and when you are cooking.

Salt Cravings

Take a cucumber (the serving size depends on your *Weight Loss Program*), peel it, and slice it into $1/4$ inch pieces. Place the slices in a container and add vinegar, salt, and pepper to taste. This serves as a crunchy, salty substitute for chips, pretzels, or popcorn.

You may also put a small amount of salt on the tip of your tongue to help stop a salt craving.

Sweet Cravings

Slice strawberries (the serving size depends on your *Weight Loss Program*) into $1/4$ inch pieces. Place the slices in a container and add Equal® or Splenda®. Let them sit at least one hour in order to get extra sweet before eating.

Peel an apple (the serving size depends on your *Weight Loss Program*), and slice it into $1/4$ inch pieces. Place the slices in a container and sprinkle cinnamon and Equal® or Splenda® between the slices. Microwave for about 1 minute or until soft for a baked apple.

Chocolate Cravings

You may try baker's chocolate or unsweetened chocolate, found near the flour and sugar section of the grocery store, and sprinkle Equal® or Splenda® on the pieces. This by no means tastes like milk chocolate, but it may help to satisfy a chocolate craving.

Starch Cravings

A starch craving usually is the desire to have something a little heavier in your stomach. For the Snack option of your *Weight Loss Program*, use turkey breast slices rolled around lettuce and dipped into fat-free salad dressing or mustard.

Bad Breath

For bad breath you may use sugar free gum, sugar free breath mints, sugar free breath sprays, or sugar free breath strips.

Constipation

Are you constipated or are you not having a bowel movement as frequently as you did before you started the *Weight Loss Program*?

If it is a timing issue and you do not feel constipated, then you do not need to be concerned. You are not eating the same as you were before the *Weight Loss Program*–less in equals less out.

If you are constipated, or having a hard painful bowel movement, then you may use a mild laxative. If no relief comes in two days, then you may try an enema. If constipation exists for more than 10 days, contact your primary physician.

Do not use the so-called colon scrubbers, internal cleansers, strong herbal teas, powders, and pills meant to clean out the large intestine (also known as the colon or bowel), without first talking to your primary physician.

Diarrhea and Gas

Diarrhea and gas can occur if you are eating more leafy green vegetables than usual. The treatment is to decrease the amounts of those vegetables. You may use any preparation containing simethicone to fight gas.

What to Do When You Have a Cold

♦ Avoid all cough syrups except Robitussin DM®.

♦ Avoid all throat lozenges and cough drops except those that are sugar free. Most of them have as much sugar as candy. If you need something else to soothe your throat, use an anesthetic spray such as Chloraseptic Spray®. You may also gargle with warm salt water, but not with other commercial gargle preparations.

♦ Avoid all cold tablets except those that say *non-drowsy* on the package.

♦ While you are sick you may take 500 milligrams of vitamin C (ascorbic acid) up to 4 times a day.

♦ It is not necessary to drink fruit juices or eat soups when you have a cold or flu. You can get the same benefits from a loving hug, lots of water, sugar free sodas, and other calorie-free liquids.

♦ Never use whiskey, honey, vinegar, or a combination as a cough medicine. This will wreck your diet and not really help. The same goes for peppermint and other hard candies.

♦ If you require medical treatment, show these instructions to your doctor.

♦ Avoid prolonged use of nasal sprays and inhalers as they usually cease to work after three or four days.

♦ Most importantly – sick people belong home in the bed!

Going on Vacation

Vacations are often contemplated with ambivalent feelings of pleasure and apprehension when you have weight problems. Yet, by increasing your awareness of potential problems and planning to overcome them, there is no reason why you should not enjoy a well-earned vacation.

The late Dr. Peter Lindner, a respected weight loss expert and one of my mentors, has stated,

> *"Your attitude is most important. A change of scenery must not be viewed as an excuse for abandoning the program, nor as an invitation to reward yourself for weight reduction accomplishments achieved at home. Instead, it should be regarded as an opportunity to learn and practice new skills of weight control. It might even be considered to be an exciting challenge to achieve the goal of enjoying yourself to the utmost, while still maintaining sensible eating and activity habits."*

While away, give yourself lots of pleasures other than eating, such as taking brisk walks through interesting places and along the shore. Such enjoyable pastimes are not only invigorating, but also help to tone up your muscles and to release pleasure-providing chemical substances called "endorphins." By doing this, you are likely to return from your vacation feeling fitter and looking slimmer than before you left home.

Create a strong mental image of how unpleasant it would be to return home to a scale that tells you that you weigh more than before you left. At that stage, your vacation will be over and all you will have is a more overweight body. On the other hand, if you weigh less when you return, then obviously you will feel much happier and your vacation will have achieved something, rather than ruining the top priority in your life at the moment which is to reach and maintain your healthy weight.

Prepare for the plane, car, train, or boat trip by having an appropriate meal prior to departure. Hotel rooms and holiday condos should be fat-proofed. In other words, keep all forbidden foods away. Relieved of the customary daily stresses, a false feeling of confidence might lead to a belief that "a few extra mouthfuls can't hurt."

This is not true. Remember that deviating from your *Weight Loss Program* may cause you to store fat rather than mobilize or break it down. Be particularly careful of exotic or native drinks or food concoctions. Remember, "When in doubt as to whether it's allowed or not, leave it out."

Make sure you drink lots of W-A-T-E-R even if you have to carry it in a flask with you or even if you have to buy it because the local tap water is unsafe.

Your vacations will be much more enjoyable if you do not allow yourself to ruin your weight reduction program. For instance, your plane seat will be more comfortable, and you will have much more energy to enjoy all the wonderful sights and experiences of your vacation. Plus, you will be proud and much less self-conscious to show off your new bikini. You will feel more confident meeting new people and you will have a good excuse to buy new clothes for your next vacation as your old ones become too big for you.

Keep in Mind

♦ Learn from your past experiences. If you have gained weight on vacation in the past, try to prevent the factors that caused this.

♦ Be assertive with any host and make sure they do not talk you into eating anything that is not on your *Weight Loss Program.*

♦ Finally, remember that as human beings, none of us is perfect. Do the best you can under the circumstances, and if you do make any mistakes, do not feel that you might as well make more. This is not true. Get right back on your *Weight Loss Program* without delay. Shortening the period between the deviations and resuming your program is one of the secrets of success in weight reduction.

Preplanning, common sense, motivation, and a bit of self-control in applying the principles that have been taught can make your vacation a wonderful experience and, most importantly, a slimming experience.

Holidays, Birthdays, Anniversaries

This section covers how to deal with Christmas day, Thanksgiving day, Easter day, your birthday, and your anniversary. In other words, just the "day," not the entire weekend. To keep the scale from going up, make wise choices and keep your portions small. You can still enjoy the day tasting your favorite foods. Just make sure it is only a taste. Have more vegetables than starch, have one dessert instead of two, alternate a sparkling mineral water or diet soda with each cocktail. The day after Christmas, the day after Thanksgiving, the day after Easter, the day after your birthday, and the day after your anniversary, get right back on track with your *Weight Loss Program.*

Be Aware of the Feeder

A "feeder" is anyone who tempts, encourages, or badgers you to go off your *Weight Loss Program*. Some feeders may not even realize that they are, in fact, a feeder. Regardless of their intention, the results unfortunately are the same: you stop following your *Weight Loss Program*.

Some of their tactics may be direct while others are very subtle. Common examples include:

- Inviting you to their home for dinner when they have nothing you can eat without going off your diet;

- Making you feel guilty about not eating with the group anymore; and

- Always suggesting the activity of going out to eat instead of another alternative.

Be aware of the feeders in your life, the reasons for their sabotage, and the best ways to handle their actions.

We use feminine descriptions here, but males can be feeders as well.

The Thin Feeder

She may be of normal weight or slightly overweight, but she always looks thinner standing next to you. She also usually gets all of the attention. Now that you are losing weight, you are beginning to get all of the attention and she may not like it.

The Overweight Feeder

She has battled being overweight just like you. But at this point she has tried so many diets that she has given up and decided to remain at an unhealthy weight. You were eating buddies. It is sometimes easier to overeat when everyone else at the table is overeating as well. Now that you are no longer going to get ice cream or going to the all-you-can-eat buffet, she may miss that time you spent together. Or, even worse, she may feel that you now think you are better than she.

The Grandmother-Figure Feeder

She does not have to be your grandmother, but she shows love by feeding you. She thinks all this stuff about being obese is ridiculous. She grew up in the country and has been overweight all her life, but she is still on God's great earth. "Only fruit for breakfast? That's hogwash. You need something to stick to your bones like biscuits and gravy."

What to Do

With all of these feeders, first determine their intention. Do they really care about you or is jealousy beginning to creep into your relationship?

For those who are genuine, explain to them that you are trying to get to a healthy weight and that you will feel much better mentally and physically once you reach your goal. Let them know that you need their support while you are on this journey. Suggest alternatives instead of eating activities. For the grandmother-figure, though, sometimes you just have to eat what she prepares in order to spare her feelings. Get right back on your diet when you return to your own environment.

For those who are not genuine, re-evaluate the role they play in your life. People who knowingly try to get you off your diet are not your true friends, nor do they have your best interest at heart. Put them behind you and stay away from them as much as possible. Find others to fill the gap, true friends who will help, support, and encourage you to reach your goal.

Everyone Says I'm Beginning to Look Too Skinny

When you are losing weight, you will eventually start receiving comments from those who know you or at least saw you at your original weight. The positive comments are encouraging and will help you stay focused. However, you may receive comments that are negative and even confusing such as, "You are beginning to look too skinny" or "You look anorexic." Unless you get a comment like that from a stranger on the street, it probably comes from the fact that people are used to seeing you a certain way.

Sometimes people may even have used your being overweight to their advantage. If you started out at 240 pounds and have worked hard to get to 200 pounds, you will look different and you will get attention from those who have noticed your progress.

Before abandoning your diet at 200 pounds based on what others say, try to understand why someone would make negative comments. Are you taking attention away from the person who used to get all of the attention? Are you getting compliments now, but before no one really said anything positive about your appearance? Are you no longer eating the way those around you still eat, so they want you to feel bad or they do not want you around them any longer?

Talk to your people and remind them that you are losing weight for health reasons. Explain to them how much better you already feel in terms of your energy, your breathing, your sleeping, and just your general well-being. Let them know that you need their encouragement to reach your goal.

Walking–the Best Exercise

Walking on a treadmill, in your neighborhood, around the track, at the park or at the mall, (depending on weather and safety conditions) is the best exercise to help you tone while you are losing weight. Engaging in vigorous exercise such as running, lifting weights, stair climbing, high impact aerobics, or riding a bicycle is especially dangerous if you are obese.

Walking is easier on your joints and leads to fewer injuries than running or jogging. Health risks aside, vigorous exercise can build too much muscle. You may notice that you are getting firm, but that you are also getting bulky. Most Black women, based on their genetic makeup, are unable to engage in heavy exercise and lose all of their excess weight at the same time.

If you are bored when you walk, try listening to music or a book on tape. When walking, make sure to wear good walking shoes and loose-fitting clothing for maximum comfort.

Benefits of Walking

- Walking is an overall aerobic exercise that can help lower your blood pressure, strengthen your heart, improve your circulation, and improve your overall fitness.

- Walking is a good way to help you feel better, tone your muscles, and reduce your desire for food.

- Walking with a partner is fun and motivating. A partner can help you keep walking as part of your lifestyle.

- Walking is an inexpensive way to add physical activity to your lifestyle because you do not have to join the gym.

I Do Not Have Time to Exercise

The foods on the *Weight Loss Program* actually help you lose the weight, it is not exercise. If you have a tight schedule, given the choice between exercise and preparing a proper meal, choose preparing the proper meal.

Benefits of Working with a Bariatric Physician

What Is a Bariatric Physician?

A bariatric physician is a licensed physician (Doctor of Medicine [MD] or Doctor of Osteopathy [DO]) who, as a member of the American Society of Bariatric Physicians (ASBP), has received special training in bariatric medicine–the medical treatment of overweight, obesity and associated conditions. Bariatric physicians address overweight and obese patients with a comprehensive program of diet and nutrition, exercise, lifestyle changes and, when indicated, prescriptions for appetite suppressants and other appropriate medications. The word "bariatric" stems from the Greek word *barros*, which translates as heavy or large.

Any licensed physician can offer a medical weight loss program to patients. However, members of the ASBP have been exposed, through an extensive continuing medical education program, to specialized knowledge, tools, and techniques to enable them to design specialized medical weight loss programs tailored to the needs of individual patients. Bariatric physicians may also modify the programs, if needed, as the treatment progresses. ASBP members are uniquely equipped to treat overweight, obesity, and associated conditions.

Safe Weight Loss with a Bariatric Physician

A physician-supervised medical weight loss program is the safest and wisest way to lose weight and maintain the loss. Overweight and obesity are frequently accompanied by other medical conditions, such as type 2 diabetes, hypertension, cancer, and others. A bariatric physician is trained to diagnose and treat these conditions, which might go undetected and untreated in a non-medical weight loss program.

The physician should perform a complete medical screening including a physical exam, blood tests, electrocardiogram (EKG), blood pressure reading, urinalysis, and a medical history review.

Once the physician has reviewed the results of your complete medical screening, he or she will be able to put you on our weight reduction programs. These programs include a prescription for appetite suppressants and vitamin B12 injections.

The physician must monitor your blood pressure and weight on a regular basis. You will also receive regularly scheduled counseling sessions to discuss the particular challenges you encounter while trying to lose weight.

However, even with the addition of appetite suppressants and vitamin B12 injections, if you do not follow the prescribed weight loss program, you will not lose weight. You cannot take pills, eat whatever you want, and lose weight. It all works together.

Diet Pills

Appetite suppressants or diet pills are a very important aid in your *Weight Loss Program* if you are medically qualified to take them. However, you can take diet pills only when they are prescribed by a physician who is monitoring you on a weekly or bi-weekly schedule while you are on the program. If you are not medically suited for diet pills or if you cannot find a physician to monitor you, then you cannot take them.

The only two diet pills that I consider safe enough to give my patients are phentermine starting at 15mg per day and phendimetrazine starting at 35mg per day. Phentermine should never exceed a 30mg per day dose and phendimetrazine should never exceed 105mg per day.

You can lose weight without diet pills, but it is more difficult. However, you have the ability to do something difficult especially when the results are very important to your life and health.

Locating a Bariatric Physician

In D.C., Baltimore, and Richmond contact:

Robert S. Beale, Jr., M.D.
1712 I Street, NW
Suite 604
Washington, DC 20006
Phone: 202-463-7872
Website: www.docbeale.com

In Atlanta and Albany, Georgia contact:

J. Tom Cooper, M.D.
1234 Powers Ferry Road
Suite 104
Marietta, GA 30067
Phone (Atlanta): 770-952-7681
Phone (Albany): 229-439-0904

In Detroit, Michigan contact:

> Bill Nagler, M.D.
> 16311 Middlebelt Road
> Livonia, MI 48154
> Phone: 734-422-8040

In New York, New York contact:

> Gary Zisk, D.O.
> 8223 Bay Parkway
> Brooklyn, NY 11214
> Phone: 718-259-1979

For physicians in other areas contact the American Society of Bariatric Physicians on the Web at www.asbp.org or by phone at 303-770-2526.

Physician Warning Signs

Be very cautious of a physician who is treating you for obesity if:

- The physician does not perform a complete medical screening.

- The physician gives every patient essentially the same diet and the same pills.

- The physician prescribes diet pills, but does not monitor your blood pressure on a regular basis.

- The physician is not available to discuss your concerns and questions.

- The physician does not tell you how to contact him or her if you have side effects.

- ◆ The physician does not require you to come in for a consultation on a regular basis.

- ◆ The physician is obese.

Bariatric Surgery

Bariatric surgery has received widespread media coverage and notoriety in recent years. Gastrointestinal surgery, in particular, consists of restricting food intake by creating a small pouch at the top of the stomach with a small outlet that delays food moving out of the pouch, thereby causing a feeling of fullness. A person can eat only one-half to one cup of food without discomfort or nausea.

Potential candidates for bariatric surgery are patients with a BMI over 40. Psychological testing and analysis are often performed on the patient prior to surgery. After surgery the patient receives close nutritional monitoring during rapid weight loss and lifelong medical surveillance after surgical therapy.

The benefit is that most patients rapidly lose weight. However, some patients regain all of the lost weight within two years if they do not follow a maintenance plan.

The inherent risks with surgery become even more considerable when a patient is obese. Specific risks with gastrointestinal surgery include DEATH, abdominal hernias, gallstones, enlarging of stomach outlets, nutritional deficiencies, osteoporosis, or metabolic bone disease. Side effects may include nausea, vomiting, bowel restriction, diarrhea, dehydration, and anemia. Bariatric surgery also changes the body's biochemistry, the effects of which have not been fully researched.

You should thoroughly exhaust all other reasonable avenues of weight loss before selecting surgery. Undergoing bariatric surgery is too extreme if you have not tried everything else first and failed to lose weight. Two of the more popular bariatric surgeries are gastric banding and gastric bypass.

Gastric Banding

Adjustable gastric banding, commonly known as The LAP-BAND®, is a flexible silicone band (much like a belt buckle) placed around the top part of the stomach. The inner surface of the band is lined with an inflatable balloon that is connected to a reservoir by tubing. The balloon can be filled with water by injecting the reservoir to make the band tighter around the stomach. The band works by decreasing the amount of food the patient can eat at one time. The adjustability of the band allows the surgeon some level of control over the patient's weight loss. The amount of stomach above the band can hold approximately 20 to 25ml.

Gastric Bypass

Gastric bypass surgery reduces the capacity of the stomach to only 30cc (equivalent to two tablespoons) by stapling across the stomach with a special metal device. Thus, approximately 90% of the stomach is below the staple line and is, therefore, isolated from the passage of food through the stomach. A length of small intestine (typically 50-100cm) is stapled to the stomach above the staple line so that food passes from the 30cc gastric pouch directly into the small intestine. The severely reduced size of the stomach–in combination with the narrow diameter (1cm) of the connection between the gastric pouch and the small intestine–are responsible for significant limitations placed on the patient's ability to eat large meals after the operation.

IRS Permits Deduction of Weight Loss Programs

You can deduct the cost of your weight loss program as a medical expense. The IRS has revised its policy to give tax relief to many of you who pay out-of-pocket for your weight loss program.

You may deduct medical expenses in excess of 7.5% of your adjusted gross income. The policy, which appears in IRS Publication 502, assists taxpayers who itemize medical deductions or employees who have a medical savings account (MSA) or a flexible savings account (FSA) with their employers.

Items such as health club dues, over-the-counter products, and nutritional supplements from a health food store are not included.

Products and the treatment recommended by a bariatric physician are deductible. If you have not been keeping track of these expenses, you may request an itemized statement from your physician which you can give to your accountant to help you with this process.

Listing any of these conditions on your statement will expedite approval by IRS: cancer, cardiovascular disease, chronic venous insufficiency, daytime sleepiness, deep vein thrombosis, gallbladder disease, gout, heat disorders, high cholesterol, hypertension, impaired immune response, impaired respiratory function, infertility, liver disease, low back pain, gynecological complications, back pain, sleep apnea, stroke, diabetes type 2, urinary stress incontinence, osteoarthritis, and rheumatoid arthritis.

Do not list any conditions or diseases that you do not have.

American Society of Bariatric Physicians' Position Statement on Ephedra

"Ephedra, or ma huang, is not a single substance but rather a combination of the following six alkaloids: ephedrine, pseudoephedrine, norephedrine, norpseudoephedrine, N-methylephedrine, and N-methylpseudoephedrine. Ephedra has been used in Chinese medicine as a treatment for acute respiratory symptoms such as colds, bronchitis, or asthma. Its use was limited to several days as patients usually experienced a rapid improvement and/or resolution of their symptoms. Ephedrine and pseudoephedrine, two of the ephedra alkaloids, can stimulate receptors in the lung, cardiovascular, and central nervous systems. Ephedrine is also noted to have thermogenic or fat-burning effects.

The food supplement business, currently a $19 billion industry, capitalized on these properties to use ephedra as their 'magic weight loss elixir.' Ephedra's popularity as a weight loss agent has exponentially increased over the past decade, but so have reports of its serious and adverse side effects. The DSHEA Act of 1994 stripped the FDA of the ability to regulate the food supplement industry. As a result, no manufacturer is held to specific controls that govern the quality, purity, or concentration of products contained in supplements. A tremendous variation exists in the concentration of active alkaloids in ephedra manufactured by different companies.

Reports of serious side effects linked to the use of ephedra continue to escalate. Ephedra was implicated in the death of Baltimore Orioles pitcher Steve Bechler. On March 7, 2003, the FDA unveiled an extensive list of rules to govern the quality of dietary supplements. These rules would permit the FDA to remove products that contain contaminants or concentrations other than stated on the labeling. Enforcement of these rules may take 36 months to implement.

The American Society of Bariatric Physicians does not support or endorse the unregulated use of ephedra, or ephedra-containing products because of the documented dangers of these products."

Diet Pills from the Internet

Under no circumstances should you obtain a prescription for appetite suppressants over the Internet. In addition, many of the over-the-counter diet aids may increase your blood pressure which could be very dangerous. Do not treat yourself with prescriptions and diet aids without consulting with your medical doctor since you may seriously endanger your health.

If you obtain diet pills from the Internet or from a non-physician, you are committing a crime (illegally obtaining controlled drugs) and, even worse, you are seriously jeopardizing your life. You should never take diet pills from an illegal source, nor should you take any herbs or herbal products to aid in appetite control or to boost energy. They are usually either ineffective or dangerous.

Common Mistakes

While you are not a dieting machine and not perfect all of the time, here are some common mistakes to be aware of as you follow the *Weight Loss Program*.

1. **Believing that going off the *Weight Loss Program* just a little bit does not matter.** It is the specific foods and meals of the *Weight Loss Programs* that allow you to lose weight. Eating anything else will either slow down your progress or, even worse, cause you to gain weight.

2. **Not drinking enough water. You *must* drink two to three quarts of water per day.** Water helps your body digest food more efficiently, water suppresses the appetite naturally, and water helps your body metabolize stored fat. If you do not drink enough water your body metabolizes the fat slower, causing your weight loss to slow down.

3. **Believing that exercise makes up for not following the *Weight Loss Program*.** It is the specific foods and meals of the *Weight Loss Programs* that allow you to lose weight, not exercise. Exercise helps you to tone while you are losing weight, but exercise does not "make up" or "cancel out" eating something that is not on the *Weight Loss Program*.

4. **Believing the "X Number of Calories Burned" data on exercise machines.** Those machines factor time, distance and sometimes weight; however, they cannot tell anything else physically about who is on the machine. For example, the muscle mass of a 160 pound athlete is very different from the muscle mass of a 160 pound woman who just started instituting an exercise program for the first time in her life. Obviously they burn a different number of calories, but according to the machine, the number may be the same.

5. **Believing people when they make negative comments about your losing weight.** Until you get as close to the "Healthy Weight" BMI range as possible, you *must* continue to follow the *Weight Loss Program*. The primary concern of obesity is one of health and not one of appearance. Do not let anyone else's insecurities keep you from reaching your goal.

6. **Losing weight to your goal, or even close to your goal, and then not following the *Maintenance Program*.** You *must* follow the *Maintenance Program* or your weight will go back up. Your body always wants to grow back to its natural state. You must maintain your weight just like you maintain your hair, your nails, and your teeth.

7. **Believing that the following "healthy" foods are okay to eat while on the *Weight Loss Program*, even though they are not on the Allowed Foods list.** You will not reach your goal eating these foods. Having the words "fat-free," "low-fat," "lean" or "lite," as in "low-fat sour cream," still does not make these foods okay to eat.

DO NOT EAT:

- Applesause
- Beef
- Cereal
- Chicken thighs
- Cottage cheese
- Fruit cups
- Eggs or egg whites
- Low-fat cheese
- Low-salt crackers
- Non-dairy creamer
- Oatmeal
- Pickles
- Potatoes
- Raisins
- Skim milk
- Sour cream
- Sunflower seeds
- Turkey burgers
- Turkey sausages
- Turkey wings
- Wheat bread
- Lowfat milk
- Beans
- Brown rice
- Chicken legs
- Chicken wings
- Fat-free cookies
- Ground turkey
- Juice
- Low-fat salad dressing
- Meal replacement bars
- Nuts
- Olive oil
- Popcorn
- Frozen meals
- Rice cakes
- Soup
- Soy sauce
- Turkey bacon
- Turkey necks
- Turkey thighs
- Veggie burgers
- Yogurt
- Regular salad dressing

Five

Maintenance Program

C ongtratulations! You have worked diligently and you have reached your goal. The hard part is over. While you were following the *Weight Loss Program*, you were forcing your body to use your fat as a source of energy. It hates that, your body would rather live off of food instead of its own tissue. This is no longer necessary since you are not trying to lose any more weight. The goal is to not make any *new* fat. You will be able to enjoy your favorite foods. As with most things in life, though, it is all about moderation.

Maintaining your weight will be similar to maintaining your hair. Even though your hair looks nice and is healthy when you leave the salon, you know that it always wants to grow back to its "natural" state. You follow a certain plan in order to maintain your hair. Just so, even though you have reached your goal weight, your body always wants to grow back to its "natural" state.

You must follow the *Maintenance Program* in order to maintain your weight.

- ◆ You do not have to get a relaxer every day. You will not have to "diet" every day.

♦ You look in the mirror every day to check your hair. You will get on the scale every day to check your weight.

♦ Sometimes your hair needs a little extra treatment such as a deep conditioner because you have been swimming. Sometimes your weight may need a little extra treatment because you have been vacationing in the Bahamas for a week.

Instructions

The *Maintenance Program* is relatively simple and will not take much effort. Some of the instructions may not seem to make sense, but please follow them anyhow. If you do not, you might eventually regain all of your weight back, plus interest. If you follow the instructions, you can expect more success and less disappointment over the long haul. The *Maintenance Program* will ensure that all of the time and hard work you invested is not lost.

♦ Beginning tomorrow when you arise to start your day, you are to weigh yourself in the nude and with an empty bladder. This initial weight is your "Base Weight" and should be written down on several pieces of paper. Attach one paper to the scale, as well as several locations in your home, to avoid losing it.

♦ Weigh yourself everyday. You will no longer weigh yourself only once per week as you did when you were on the *Weight Loss Program*. By weighing yourself in a standard way, you can tell how you are progressing which will help you remain at your goal weight.

♦ On the days that the scale's position is at your Base Weight or less, you may eat whatever you wish, within reason.

♦ On the days that the scale is even a fraction of a pound over your Base Weight, follow your current *Weight Loss Program* for that day.

Here is the reason: If the scale goes up a pound or two in 24 hours, it is mostly fluid. If you follow your *Weight Loss Program*, then most of it will go away in a day or two. The danger of possibly making new fat increases if you do not weight yourself every day. If you have not weighed yourself in four days and the scale is up two pounds, then it is most likely new fat as opposed to fluid, and fat is much harder to lose.

To reiterate: **Weigh Yourself Every Day**.

◆ Keep drinking two to three quarts of water per day.

◆ Continue your usual pattern of exercise and other physical activities with no change from the way you did on the premaintenance part of your *Weight Loss Program*.

Weight Maintaining Strategies

You have worked so hard to reach your goal. Here are suggestions that will help you maintain your goal weight, but still enable you to enjoy the foods you deprived yourself of while you were following your *Weight Loss Program*.

◆ If a meal is not exciting, do not make it exciting. In other words, if nothing special is happening for lunch on Monday, you might as well have a chicken breast salad with fat-free dressing and an apple. No need to have a sandwich and chips. If nothing special is happening for dinner on Tuesday, you might as well have salmon, broccoli, and grapes instead of spaghetti and meatballs.

This way, when you are out with friends, at a social engagement, at brunch, or on vacation, you can really enjoy yourself, including being able to have dessert.

On the other hand, if you start drinking juice, hot chocolate, and regular soda, and eating oatmeal, rice, and chips every day, then you will not have as much freedom when it comes to the fun times. And, the possibility of the scale going up may become a daily battle.

- If you have a special event coming up, follow your *Weight Loss Program* a few days before the event.

- Split a large pizza with three friends.

- Nibble nuts one at a time.

- Read a book with both hands.

- Fill your desk candy dish with paper clips.

- Throw out stale potato chips.

- Counteract a mid-afternoon slump with a walk instead of cookies.

- Warm up after skiing with black coffee instead of hot chocolate.

- Try all the salads at the buffet, leaving room only for one dessert.

- Get into such interesting conversations at cocktail parties that you never quite work your way over to the hors d'oeuvre table.

- Bring four cookies into the TV room instead of the whole box.

- Have no compulsion to keep the candy dish symmetrical by reducing the jelly beans to an equal number of each color.

Final Thoughts

We wrote *The Black Diet Doctor's Solution for Black Women* out of a sincere desire to help Black women reach and maintain a healthy weight. We would be delighted to hear from our readers. Share your success stories with us. Tell us what sections were particularly helpful and how you implemented the *Weight Loss Program* and the *Maintenance Program* in your own life. Let us know the challenges you still encounter.

Fat is killing you, our Black women, often through no fault of your own. Until now, you have not been exposed to the knowledge, information, and techniques you need to lose and control your weight. This book is the solution. By following these programs, you can control your weight and, therefore, be healthier and live a longer, more productive life.

Robert S. Beale, Jr., M.D. and Lisa M. Beale
Phone: 866-211-DIET
Fax: 202-478-0686
Website: www.TheDietSolutions.com
Email: authors@TheDietSolutions.com

Appendix A

A NOTE TO YOUR SPOUSE

Y our support is sincerely needed and requested to help your spouse reach her goal of a healthy weight. Please read, consider, and apply the following suggestions as the best way to guide your spouse along her journey. All of the suggestions might not be pertinent, but some of them will be useful in giving you some guidance for being more supportive.

These remarks are offered strictly in a constructive and suggestive manner. The intent is to provide as much assistance as possible with the challenges your spouse will be facing during her weight control efforts.

Your spouse needs to get to a healthy weight. The primary concern of obesity is one of health and not one of appearance. There are too many health consequences including premature death, heart disease, diabetes, cancer, breathing problems, arthritis, stroke, and reproductive complications for her to remain overweight and obese.

You may have gotten fed up with your spouse's being heavy. You may have gotten fed up with yet another diet that your spouse will attempt to follow. One of the purposes of these suggestions is to try to avoid similar results and improve your spouse's chances of being successful this time.

◆ Try not to be a "Weight Control Policeman," even though you may have the best intentions. Your spouse may react negatively, causing her to feel guilty and rebellious, leading to overeating in private and bingeing. She is not a dieting machine, you do not want her to feel bad for going off of her diet. Instead, encourage her to not focus on what happened in the past and to refocus on the present.

◆ If you are not following a diet plan yourself, be sensitive to what you eat in front of her and what foods you bring into your home. While this is a problem for you, it helps to keep those food temptations out of her face.

◆ Suggest going for a walk with your spouse, especially if she has had a busy day or is stressed. You will be helping her to "get away" and she will be engaging in exercise. In addition, this allows you to spend more time together as a couple or as a family.

◆ If your spouse makes specific requests such as avoiding certain restaurants or certain social functions, try to oblige. She will not be on a diet forever. Making it easier for her to avoid these temptations while she is following her diet will help her weight loss tremendously.

◆ Your most valuable contribution is sincere and genuine support. Give her praise and reinforcement, letting her know that you are with her on her journey to reach a healthy weight. This can be a hug, a touch, or simply a properly-timed smile.

Appendix B

RECIPES

Suggested Items for Your Culinary Success

T hese recipes are among our favorites. All include only the foods on the *Weight Loss Programs*; therefore, they contain absolutely zero oil. Taste and presentation are extremely important, so having the proper utensils and spices is paramount. There are many references to specific kitchen items you will need. Please make the effort to acquire the following items:

- ◆ Stainless steel skillets (non-stick may also be used) (12" or 14", and 8" or 10")
  Stainless steel cookware is preferred primarily because the steel conducts heat evenly through the surface. Ease of clean-up is a must. When cooking with stainless steel, if anything should burn or stick in the bottom, simply add enough water to cover and bring to a low simmer. Scrape the bottom of the pan with a wooden or rubber spatula or spoon (never use metal). Wash in sudsy water and dry immediately.

- Stainless steel stockpot (8-quart)

- Glass baking dishes (rectangular)
  Choose a brand of bakeware that is durable sturdy and can withstand the dishwasher, moving, cooking, storing, and all wear and tear. This makes it simple for transferring your dishes from the oven for baking, to the table for serving, and then to the refrigerator for storing.

- Roasting pan

- Food processor or blender

- Kitchen timer

- Basting brush

- Measuring cup (preferably glass for easier reading)

- Measuring spoons

- Bamboo steamer

- Rubber or wood spatulas (large and small)

- Tongs

- Ladle

- Large slotted spoon

- Mortar and pestal (for grinding dry ingredients)

- Mixing bowls (set of 4)

- Wire whisks (small and large)

- Knives (good knives make cutting less of a chore)

- Cheesecloth

- Kitchen twine

- Aluminum foil

- Wire sieve (for straining)

- Colander (for draining)

- Chopping board

- Cooking sheet

- Skewers

- Air tight jars (small and large for storage)

- Spices

Probably the most important investment you will make is in the spices. Please, please, please invest in a basic spice set to get started and always try to use fresh whenever available. As your budget allows, add more spices and experiment with the flavors.

Notes on Recipes

- "Sweetener" may be Equal® or Splenda®, not sugar.

- "Cooking spray" must be fat-free.

- Unless noted, each recipe may be used for all of the *Weight Loss Programs*.

- Adjust serving sizes based on your *Weight Loss Program*.

DRIZZLES & GLAZES

Great for drizzling over salads, meats or fruit.

Vinaigrette

2   cloves garlic
4   tablespoons Dijon-style mustard
1   teaspoon fresh lemon juice
1   cup balsamic vinegar
1   heaping teaspoon basil, fresh
    salt
    ground black pepper

Chop the garlic and crush it into a paste in a small bowl with the bottom side of a spoon or in a mortar. Whisk together the mustard, lemon juice, and vinegar in a small bowl. Add the garlic and basil. Salt and pepper to taste. Use lemon for garnish.

Strawberry (excellent with poultry)

1   pound strawberries
    sweetener to taste

Pour enough water to cover the strawberries in the bottom of a saucepan by 1 inch. Bring to a slow simmer and cook for about 20 minutes. Stir every few minutes to keep the sauce from sticking. Taste the sauce and add sweetener as desired. Sauce can be allowed to cool or can be served as is. For a smooth sauce, strain through a sieve. Garnish with sliced strawberries.

Apple or Pear Coulis (excellent with poultry)

3   medium apples
or
3   medium pears
$\frac{1}{2}$ lemon, fresh

Peel and core the fruit and rub the cut sides with half a lemon. Cover them with water and cook until soft in a saucepan. Puree them or force through a strainer with a ladle or large wooden spoon. Sweeten to taste.

Mustard glaze (excellent with poultry)

4   tablespoons Dijon-style mustard
2   tablespoons fresh lemon juice
4   cloves garlic, peeled and minced
1   tablespoon fresh ginger, minced
1   teaspoon dried thyme
1   teaspoon ground black pepper
    salt to taste

Combine ingredients in a food processor and blend until smooth. Brush on all sides of meat before and during cooking. Remaining may be drizzled as a garnish or used for dipping.

SALSAS, SAUCES & CHUTNEYS

Fruit Salsa (especially good with chicken and fish)

$1/2$ cup green apple, diced
$1/2$ cup pear, diced
$1/3$ cup green bell pepper, diced
$1/3$ cup red bell pepper, diced
2   tablespoons rice vinegar
1   packet sweetener
1   tablespoon cilantro, minced
$1/4$ teaspoon crushed red pepper

Combine apple, pear, bell peppers, vinegar, sweetener, cilantro and crushed red peppers in a large bowl. Best when served immediately or cover and refrigerate.

Tangerine Chutney (an excellent glaze for chicken and turkey)

5   tangerines
1   teaspoon cumin, ground
$1/4$ teaspoon white pepper

In a small saucepan, squeeze the juice of 2 tangerines. Cook over medium heat. Peel and section the remaining 3 tangerines. On a cutting board, slice the tangerine segments in half and mash with the backside of a spoon; add to saucepan. Whisk in cumin and white pepper. Continue to cook, stirring until slightly thickened.

Green Chutney (excellent with steamed fish)

$1^{1}/_{4}$ teaspoons whole cumin seed
1   small jalapeno pepper, minced
or
2-3 Thai chile peppers, minced
1   cup mint, chopped medium
2   cups cilantro, chopped medium
1   tablespoon ginger, chopped
$1^{1}/_{2}$ tablespoons garlic, chopped
1   packet sweetener
$^{1}/_{4}$ teaspoon black pepper
$1^{1}/_{2}$ teaspoons salt
1   tablespoon lime juice

In a small skillet coated with cooking spray, toast the cumin seeds over medium heat. Toss often until very fragrant, about 3 minutes. Remove from pan, let cool, then grind in a mortar or spice grinder. Transfer cumin to a bowl, add remaining ingredients, and toss well to combine.

*Can be made hotter or milder by adjusting the amount of minced peppers used.

Kimchi (a Korean spicy cabbage side dish)

$1\frac{1}{2}$ pounds Napa cabbage
4   tablespoons salt
1   cup water
4   green onions, chopped fine
4   cloves garlic, crushed
2   tablespoons ginger
1   medium onion, chopped
2   red peppers, halved, sliced thin
3   teaspoons chili powder
2   packets sweetener

Place shredded cabbage in a large mixing bowl and sprinkle evenly with salt. Mix well. Pour water over cabbage, cover, and refrigerate overnight. Drain the next day and set aside the cabbage and the reserved liquid in separate bowls. Add the green onions, garlic, ginger, onions, red peppers, chili powder, and sweetener to cabbage. Mix well, then pack the mixture into a large jar. Pour in enough of the reserved liquid to fill the jar. Cover with plastic wrap and allow it to sit for 2-3 days on a sunny windowsill or in a cupboard. Thereafter, store in the refrigerator. Mixture can be kept for several weeks.

Tomato-Basil Sauce
Weight Loss Program A Only

1   large onion, chopped
1   large carrot, chopped
1   14 oz. can Italian plum tomatoes, drained and chopped
1   large tomato, chopped
2   tablespoons fresh basil, chopped
2   tablespoons fresh oregano, chopped
1   teaspoon salt
$^1/_2$ teaspoon ground black pepper
2   teaspoons garlic, minced

Coat a large skillet with cooking spray and heat over medium heat. Add onions and carrots. Cook until 2 minutes, stirring occasionally to avoid burning. Add all remaining ingredients and cook until tender and excess liquid evaporates, about 20 minutes. In a food processor or blender, puree mixture until smooth.

COOKING STOCK

Better than using broth or bouillon.

Note: Stock is best used the day it is made, however, it may be divided and stored in air-tight containers for later use.

Vegetable Stock (excellent for cooking greens and steaming vegetables; great substitute for water)

2   large yellow onions
2   medium carrots *
1   stalk celery
4   cloves garlic, peeled
1   large bouquet garni (ingredients below)
        - 1 bay leaf, 1 small bunch fresh thyme, 1 small bunch parsley and 1 small bunch tarragon branches tied together with kitchen twine
4   quarts cold water

* Only add for Weight Loss Program A

Peel and dice the carrots, onions, and celery. Coat the bottom of an 8-quart stock pot with cooking spray and sauté the diced vegetables and garlic. Do not allow them to brown. Add the bouquet garni and cold water and bring to a simmer over medium heat. Simmer gently for 1 hour and let cool. Strain out the vegetables using a strainer or sieve.

Chicken Stock

2   large yellow onions
2   medium carrots *
1   stalk celery
4   cloves garlic, peeled
1   large bouquet garni (ingredients below)
     - 1 bay leaf, 1 small bunch fresh thyme, 1 small bunch parsley and 1 small bunch tarragon branches tied together with kitchen twine
4   quarts cold water
5   pounds chicken breasts with skin and bones

* Only add for Weight Loss Program A

Peel and dice the carrots, onions, and celery. Coat the bottom of an 8-quart stock pot with cooking spray and sauté the diced vegetables and garlic. Do not allow them to brown. Add the water and bouquet garni. Simmer over medium heat for 30 minutes.

Rinse chicken parts under cold running water. Trim excess fat off chicken parts. Add to the pot and cook slowly for about 2 hours skimming off any fat or froth that comes to the surface. Add small amounts of water as needed to keep chicken parts submerged. Strain the stock through a cheesecloth lined strainer or sieve and let cool. The next day when stock is cold, spoon off and discard any fat that has congealed on the top.

Fish Stock (great for steaming fish; great substitute for water)

5	pounds assorted fish or fish bones
1	medium onion
1	medium carrot *
$1/2$	stalk celery
1	bunch leeks, green tops only
1	clove garlic, cut crosswise
1	large bouquet garni (ingredients below)

    - 1 bay leaf, 1 small bunch fresh thyme, 1 small bunch parsley and 1 small bunch tarragon branches tied together with kitchen twine

4	quarts cold water

* *Only add for Weight Loss Program A*

A combination of fish and fish heads is best. Cut fish into 1-inch pieces. Rinse fish heads and bones under cold running water. Transfer to a colander to drain. Peel and dice the onion, carrot, and celery into small cubes. Cut leeks into 1-inch lengths.

Coat the bottom of an 8-quart stock pot with cooking spray and sauté the diced vegetables, leek greens, and garlic for 5 minutes. Add the bones and fish. Stir the ingredients over medium heat another five minutes or until the bones turn white. Add the water and bring to a gentle simmer. As the stock simmers, skim off any fat or froth that floats to the top. Add the bouquet garni. Add small amounts of water as needed to keep the fish parts submerged. Continue to simmer for another 2 hours. Strain the stock through a cheesecloth lined strainer or sieve and let cool. The next day, spoon off and discard any fat that has congealed on the top.

SALADS

Cucumber Salad

2   packets sweetener
$^3/_4$ cup white vinegar
$^3/_4$ cup water
$^3/_4$ teaspoon salt
1   tablespoon red pepper, crushed
5   large cucumbers, peeled and thinly sliced
2   small yellow onions, thinly sliced and rings separated
2   heaping tablespoons green onions, sliced

Combine sweetener, vinegar, water, salt and pepper; set aside. In a large shallow dish, place cucumbers and onion rings. Add vinegar mixture and toss gently. Cover and chill at least 3 hours before serving. Drain and discard marinade; place cucumbers and onions in a serving bowl. Garnish with green onions.

Asian Cucumber-Shrimp Salad

2   large cucumbers
1   teaspoon salt
6   tablespoons white wine vinegar
1   packet sweetener
1   tablespoon ginger, peeled and sliced thin
1   cup small shrimp, frozen and cooked

Peel cucumber and cut in half lengthwise. Scrape out and discard seeds. Cut cucumber into thin slices. Place slices in a bowl, sprinkle with $1/2$ teaspoon salt, toss and let sit at least 30 minutes. Whisk together vinegar, sweetener, and $1/2$ teaspoon salt until dry ingredients are dissolved. Drain cucumbers, pressing the slices to release all their liquid. Add sliced ginger and shrimp; pour dressing over all. Toss to mix well.

Crab Salad

$^3/_4$ cup fat-free mayonnaise
$^1/_3$ cup ketchup
$^1/_4$ teaspoon cayenne pepper
2   tablespoons green onions, chopped fine
1   tablespoon parsley, chopped fine
1   teaspoon fresh lemon juice
1   teaspoon horseradish
$^1/_4$ teaspoon salt
1   pound crab meat
$^3/_4$ cup celery, sliced thin
$^1/_2$ teaspoon celery seeds
    lettuce leaves (any kind)
1   heaping tablespoon parsley, chopped large
2   medium tomatoes, cut into wedges *
2   lemons, cut into wedges

* *Only add for Weight Loss Program A*

In a medium bowl, combine fat-free mayonnaise, ketchup, cayenne pepper, green onions, finely chopped parsley, lemon juice, horseradish, and salt; set aside. Flake the crab meat, remove shells and place in a large bowl. Stir in celery. Add $^3/_4$ cup of the dressing and toss crab mixture until well coated.

To serve, line salad plates with lettuce leaves. Divide salad and mound in the center of each plate. Garnish with tomato wedges and sprinkle with fresh parsley. Serve with lemon wedges and drizzle lightly with juice. Use remaining dressing on the side.

Tuna and Arugula Salad

4   tuna steaks, 1" thick
$1/3$ cup plus 2 tablespoons fat-free vinaigrette dressing, divided
1   large bag arugula greens
$1/2$ large red onion, thinly sliced
1   pint cherry tomatoes, halved *
    salt
    coarse black pepper

* Only add for Weight Loss Program A

Brush steaks with 2 tablespoons salad dressing; cover and refrigerate 1 hour. Heat broiler. Place steaks on broiler rack coated with cooking spray. Broil about 5 inches from heat for 10 minutes. Set aside and keep warm. Combine arugula, onion, and tomatoes in a large bowl. Heat remaining salad dressing in microwave. Pour over salad and toss well. Divide salad onto 4 plates, top with steaks. Salt and pepper to taste and serve immediately.

Spicy Shrimp and Roasted Red Pepper Salad

1   large onion, chopped
15 black peppercorns
1   small bunch plus 2 teaspoons parsley, chopped and divided
1   sliced lemon
2   tablespoons salt
1   teaspoon cayenne pepper
3   bay leaves
2   pounds jumbo shrimp, peeled and deveined, tails intact
2   large red bell peppers
2   teaspoons fresh mint
1   teaspoon fresh lemon juice
    ground black pepper to taste
1   10 oz. bag field greens lettuce mix
1   pint cherry or grape tomatoes, halved *

* *Only add for Weight Loss Program A*

In a large pot filled with 4 quarts of water, combine onion, peppercorns, parsley bunch, sliced lemon, salt, cayenne pepper and bay leaves; bring to a boil. Reduce heat, add shrimp, and simmer for 2 minutes. Drain shrimp and cool.

Preheat oven to 500 degrees. Place bell peppers in a small baking dish and roast until skin is charred and the flesh is softened, about 15-20 minutes. Set peppers aside. When cooled, remove and discard skin, stem, and seeds. Then cut flesh length-wise into $\frac{1}{4}$-inches wide strips. In a medium bowl, combine shrimp, peppers, parsley, mint, and lemon juice. Season with salt and pepper. Set aside for 30 minutes to allow flavors to develop. Serve at room temperature on a bed of lettuce. Garnish with tomatoes.

Curried Chicken or Turkey Salad

1½ cups green apples, cubed
1   teaspoon fresh lemon juice
3   cups cooked chicken breast or turkey breast, cubed
1   cup fat-free mayonnaise
1   teaspoon Dijon mustard
1   clove garlic, minced
½   teaspoon salt
½   teaspoon ground black pepper
2   tablespoons curry powder
1   stalk celery, sliced thin
    lettuce leaves
    white seedless grapes

Peel and core apples; cut into small cubes. Place apples in a medium bowl and drizzle with lemon juice to prevent browning. Add chicken, fat-free mayonnaise, mustard, garlic, salt, pepper, curry powder, and celery. Mix well. Divide salad onto plates lined with lettuce leaves. Garnish with grapes on the side.

Most Excellent Tuna Salad

2   6 oz. cans solid white tuna
3   stalks celery, diced fine
3   tablespoons fat-free mayonnaise
1   medium onion, chopped fine
2   tablespoons fresh parsley, chopped
$1/_2$ teaspoon dill, dried
$1/_4$ teaspoon black pepper
4   teaspoons capers, drained
$1/_2$ teaspoon celery seeds
$1/_4$ teaspoon fresh lemon juice
     lettuce leaves
     tomato wedges *
     salt
     ground black pepper

* Only add for Weight Loss Program A

Combine all ingredients in a bowl. Refrigerate overnight. Serve on a bed of lettuce and garnish with tomatoes. Salt and pepper to taste.

Pepper Salad

1 medium red bell pepper
1 medium green bell pepper
1 medium yellow bell pepper
2 cloves garlic, crushed
$\frac{1}{4}$ teaspoon salt
1 pinch ground red pepper
2 tablespoons apple cider vinegar

Blanch bell peppers in boiling water for 2 minutes and drain. Plunge into cold water and drain again. Combine garlic, salt and pepper to make a paste. Stir into vinegar and pour over bell peppers. Cover and chill until ready to serve.

Tangerine Spinach Salad

5 tangerines
1 small red onion
1 large bag spinach
$\frac{1}{3}$ cup cider vinegar
1 clove garlic, crushed
$\frac{1}{4}$ teaspoon salt
$\frac{1}{4}$ teaspoon coarse black pepper

In small bowl, squeeze the juice of 2 tangerines. Peel and section the remaining 3 tangerines. Cut onion in half and slice thinly. In a large bowl, combine spinach, onions and tangerine sections. To the tangerine juice, add vinegar, garlic, and salt. Whisk together and microwave for 30 seconds. Pour hot dressing over spinach mixture and toss until slightly wilted. Season with pepper and serve.

Fruit Salad

1	large grapefruit
2	medium oranges
1	medium cantaloupe *
1	pint strawberries, halved
1	bunch white seedless grapes
1	packet sweetener
1	teaspoon fresh lemon juice
	whole mint leaves

* Only add for Weight Loss Program A

Peel grapefruit and oranges. Over a large bowl, section oranges and grapefruit and remove membrane. Fruit juices should collect in the bowl. Cut cantaloupe in half and remove seeds. Using a melon baller, make uniform melon balls and add to bowl. Add strawberries and grapes. Combine sweetener and lemon juice and add to bowl. Toss everything gently and serve in dessert dishes garnished with mint leaves.

Warm Chicken or Turkey Salad with Asparagus and Ginger

1   bunch asparagus
4   boneless, skinless chicken breasts, cut into thick strips
    or
2   turkey breasts, cut into thick strips)
    salt
    coarse black pepper
1   medium red onion, peeled and sliced
2   bunches spring onions, root ends removed, white only cut into
        1" pieces
$^1/_2$ teaspoon ginger
1   bunch cilantro, chopped
1   lemon, squeeze for juice
2   bags spring lettuce mix

Cut off the ends and remove scales from asparagus spears. Blanche in boiling water for 2 minutes and drain. Plunge into cold water and drain again. Let cool, pat dry, and cut into $^1/_2$-inch pieces. Place the chicken strips in a bowl and season with salt and pepper. Coat the bottom of a large skillet with cooking spray over medium heat. Add chicken and cook until golden brown. Transfer chicken to a bowl and set aside.

To the same skillet add red onion and sauté for 2-3 minutes. Add spring onions and cook for an additional minute. Transfer onions to bowl of chicken. Combine blanched asparagus, ginger, and cilantro. Season with salt, pepper, and lemon juice. Serve warm over a bed of lettuce.

Salmon Salad

$1/4$ cup fresh lemon juice
$1/4$ cup red wine vinegar
1   clove garlic, minced
$1/4$ teaspoon oregano, dried
$1/4$ teaspoon salt
$1/4$ teaspoon ground black pepper
$1/4$ teaspoon celery seeds
$1/4$ teaspoon rosemary, dried
1   14 oz. can red salmon
     whole lettuce leaves, any kind
5   cups iceberg lettuce, chopped
1   large cucumber
2   medium tomatoes, chopped *
$1/4$ cup green onions, sliced
2   tablespoons capers, drained

* Only add for Weight Loss Program A

In a small bowl whisk together lemon juice, vinegar, garlic, oregano, salt, pepper, celery seeds, and rosemary until blended; set aside. Drain salmon, remove bones and dark skin. Break into bite-size pieces and set aside.

Line a large salad bowl with lettuce leaves and then add chopped lettuce. Peel cucumber, cut in half length-wise and slice thinly. Scatter over the chopped lettuce. Arrange the salmon on the top in the center, placing the tomatoes around the edge. Sprinkle with green onions and capers. Pour half of the dressing over salad. Serve remaining dressing on the side.

Roasted Beet Salad*
Weight Loss Program A Only

8   small beets
3   tablespoons balsamic vinegar
1   teaspoon fresh lemon juice
$1/_2$ teaspoon salt
$1/_4$ teaspoon coarse black pepper
2   small vidalia onions, sliced into thin rings
1   large head radicchio lettuce, chopped
1   heaping tablespoon fresh oregano

Preheat oven to 400 degrees. Clean and trim beets reserving greens to the side. Wrap beets in aluminum foil and place on baking sheet. Roast until tender, about 45 minutes; set aside to cool. When the beets have cooled, peel and cut into eighths. In a bowl, whisk together vinegar, lemon juice, salt and pepper. Toss the beets and onion rings in dressing. Clean the beet greens and radicchio, drain and pat dry. Chop and transfer to serving bowl. Using a slotted spoon, arrange beets and onion rings on top. Drizzle with remaining dressing and garnish with oregano.

VEGETABLES

Home style Collard Greens or Kale or Green Beans or Cabbage

1   large bunch collard greens
    or
2   pounds kale
    or
2   medium cabbages
    or
2   pounds green beans *
2   quarts vegetable stock, use recipe found in the *Cooking Stock* section
2   serrano peppers, stems removed
    salt
    ground black pepper

* Only add for Weight Loss Program A

Clean greens in warm, slightly salted water. Chop or tear into bite sized pieces. If preparing green beans, snap the ends off, snap in half, and rinse under running water in a colander. If preparing cabbage, cut in half and remove core. Cut each half in half and chop into bite size pieces. In a large pot, heat vegetable stock under medium heat. Add the greens or beans or cabbage and the peppers. Cook until tender. Salt and pepper to taste.

Sautéed Spinach with Garlic

2   cloves garlic, peeled and sliced thin lengthwise
2   pounds fresh spinach
    salt
    ground black pepper
1   medium lemon, wedged

Spray a large sauté pan with cooking spray and heat over medium heat. Add garlic and cook until golden brown, 2-3 minutes. Using a slotted spoon, transfer garlic to a paper towel and set aside. Clean and spray the sauté pan with cooking spray and heat over medium heat. Chop the spinach and add to the pan in batches. Cover and cook until spinach begins to wilt, 4-5 minutes. Transfer cooked spinach to serving bowl and season with salt and pepper to taste. Sprinkle garlic over spinach, drizzle with lemon, and serve warm. Garnish with lemon wedges.

Steamed Greens (kale, collards or other spicy green such as arugula)

2 cups vegetable stock, use recipe found in the *Cooking Stock* section
1 pound greens
  salt
  ground pepper
1 cup cherry tomatoes, halved *
1 pinch nutmeg

* Only add for Weight Loss Program A

In a large pot, bring vegetable stock to a boil. Place greens in a steamer basket, put in pot, cover, and steam until wilted; about 3 minutes. Drain. Transfer to serving bowl and add salt and pepper to taste. Garnish with tomatoes and a pinch of nutmeg.

Vegetable Stir-Fry

2   medium zucchinis, sliced
1   cup broccoli
2   cups fresh mushrooms, sliced *
$1/_2$ green bell pepper, cut into strips
$1/_2$ teaspoon ground cumin
$1/_2$ teaspoon salt
$1/_4$ teaspoon ground black pepper
1   cup tomato, chopped large *
$1/_2$ cup green onions, chopped

Only add for Weight Loss Program A

Spray wok or large skillet generously with cooking spray. Add zucchini, broccoli, mushrooms, bell peppers, cumin, salt and pepper. Cook over medium heat for 4 or 5 minutes until vegetables are crisp-tender. Add tomato and green onion and cook for 1 minute.

Marinated Asparagus

1   pound fresh asparagus
1   cup fat-free Italian dressing
1   tablespoon cider vinegar
$1/4$ teaspoon tarragon, dried
$1/4$ teaspoon basil, dried
$1/4$ teaspoon oregano, dried
$1/4$ teaspoon ground black pepper
1   clove garlic, crushed
$1/2$ red pepper, diced
    romaine lettuce

Cut off the ends and remove scales from asparagus spears. Cook in a small amount of boiling water until crisp tender. Whisk together all ingredients except lettuce. Drain asparagus and place in a food storage bag. Pour in dressing and let stand for 1 hour. Arrange lettuce in the bottom of a shallow dish. Place the asparagus on top and drizzle with remaining dressing. Garnish with diced peppers.

Lemon Carrots*
Weight Loss Program A Only

1   large bag baby carrots
1   heaping tablespoon fresh parsley
    salt

Steam carrots or cook in boiling salted water until tender, 5 to 8 minutes. Drain and transfer to serving dish. Squeeze fresh juice from lemons all over. Salt to taste. Garnish with parsley.

Vegetable Bake*
Weight Loss Program A Only

1   yellow bell pepper
1   green bell pepper
1   red bell pepper
2   red onions
2   small yellow squashes
2   small zucchinis
4   cloves garlic, peeled and thinly sliced
1   tablespoon fresh oregano, chopped
2   tablespoons fresh parsley, chopped
1   tablespoon balsamic vinegar
    salt
    ground black pepper

Preheat oven to 425 degrees. In a mixing bowl, combine all vegetables and oregano. Spread on baking sheet coated with cooking spray. Bake for 20 minutes, turning several times. Let cool slightly, then add parsley and vinegar and toss. Salt and pepper to taste.

Zesty Carrots*
Weight Loss Program A Only

4   carrots, sliced
$\frac{1}{3}$ cup fat-free mayonnaise
$\frac{1}{2}$ cup water
$1\frac{1}{2}$ tablespoons minced onions
1   tablespoon horseradish
$\frac{1}{4}$ teaspoon salt
$\frac{1}{4}$ ground black pepper

Preheat oven to 375 degrees. Coat a small baking dish with cooking spray. In a saucepan, boil carrots until just tender. Do not over cook. Drain and transfer to the baking dish and set aside. In another bowl, combine mayonnaise, water, onion, horseradish, salt and pepper. Pour over carrots, but do not stir. Bake for 15 minutes. Add salt and pepper to taste.

Steamed Brussel Sprouts*
Weight Loss Program A Only

1   pound brussel sprouts
2   teaspoons fresh thyme
1   tablespoon balsamic vinegar
$\frac{1}{4}$ teaspoon salt
$\frac{1}{4}$ teaspoon white pepper

Blanch sprouts in a pot of boiling lightly salted water or vegetable stock until tender, about 10-12 minutes. Immediately transfer to cold water bath. Cool, then drain and pat dry. Cut in half and transfer to bowl. Add thyme, vinegar, salt and pepper. Toss to coat and serve.

SEAFOOD

Crab cakes

1   teaspoon dry mustard
$1/_2$ teaspoon fresh lemon juice
$1^1/_2$ teaspoons Dijon-styled mustard
1   teaspoon fresh parsley, chopped
1   tablespoon fat-free mayonnaise
1   teaspoon Old Bay Seafood Seasoning
1   teaspoon celery seed
8   ounces crab meat, lump meat preferred
     paprika

Preheat oven to 325 degrees and spray a baking sheet with coated with cooking spray. Combine all ingredients except the crab meat in a mixing bowl. Gently fold in crab meat. Mold into evenly sized cakes and place on a baking sheet. Bake until golden brown. Dust with paprika to garnish.

Roasted Bass with Herb and Pepper Rub

$1/4$ teaspoon ground black pepper
1 teaspoon ground cumin
1 teaspoon thyme
1 teaspoon oregano, dried
1 teaspoon coriander, ground
4 striped or black bass fillets, 7 ounces each, $1/2$" thick
   salt
1 teaspoon paprika
1 heaping teaspoon green onions, sliced thin
   lemon wedges, squeeze for a little juice to drizzle

Preheat oven to 450 degrees, with the rack near the top. Combine pepper, cumin, thyme, oregano, and coriander in a small bowl. Dry the fillets with paper towels and season with salt to taste. Sprinkle herb-pepper mixture evenly over fillets and rub in gently. Coat the bottom of a roasting pan large enough to hold all the fillets comfortably. Place the fillets in the pan, skin side down, and put the pan in the oven on the top rack. Roast fillets until they are just cooked through, about 10 minutes. The flesh should be opaque and the skin should be crisped. Lift out with a spatula and place on a serving platter. Sprinkle with onions and paprika. Garnish with lemon wedges. Drizzle a little lemon juice over all.

Seared Tuna with Wasabi Mayonnaise

2   tablespoons fat-free mayonnaise
$^1/_4$ teaspoon salt
$^1/_4$ teaspoon ground black pepper
$^1/_2$ packet sweetener
2   teaspoons Wasabi paste
4   tuna steaks, 1" thick
1   lime, squeeze for juice
     radicchio lettuce leaves

In a small bowl combine mayonnaise, salt, pepper, sweetener and wasabi; set aside. Rinse steaks and pat dry. In a shallow dish, drizzle lime juice over tuna steaks; set aside 30 minutes. Heat a large skillet coated with cooking spray over high heat. Transfer steaks to skillet and sear on each side until brown. Transfer to serving platter lined with lettuce leaves and garnish generously with mayonnaise mixture.

Maryland Dungeness Crab

1   cup cider vinegar
3   tablespoons Old Bay Seasoning, divided
1   halved lemon
2   Dungeness crabs

In a large stock pot bring 4 cups of water to a rapid boil. Add vinegar and 2 tablespoons seasoning. Squeeze the lemons and add the halves to the pot. Add crabs and sprinkle with remaining seasoning. Cover tightly. Remove when crabs are bright red.

Fish & Veggie Packets

2   teaspoons garlic, minced
$1/_2$ cup green onions
2   teaspoons ginger, minced
$1/_4$ teaspoon ground black pepper
4   tilapia or any fish fillets
2   red bell peppers
2   large heads broccoli
1   large head cauliflower *

* *Only add for Weight Loss Program A*

Combine garlic, green onions, ginger, and black pepper in a small bowl. Rinse fish and pat dry. Clean and remove seeds form bell peppers. Cut florets from cauliflower and broccoli heads. Rinse and drain in a colander.

Preheat oven to 425 degrees. Cut four large squares of aluminum foil. Spray each with cooking spray. Rub each fillet with spice mixture and place a fillet in the center of each square. Divide the bell peppers and broccoli between the four squares and place on top of each fillet. Sprinkle with the scallions. Fold the sides of each square to the center and fold over the loose ends to seal. Place on a large baking sheet and bake for 10 minutes or until fish flakes easily.

Roasted Herb Salmon

4   salmon fillets, 5 ounces each, about $1\frac{1}{2}$" thick
2   tablespoons Dijon-style mustard
2   tablespoons fresh lemon juice
1   tablespoon fresh thyme, minced
    or
1   teaspoon thyme, dried
1   tablespoon fresh rosemary, minced
    or
1   teaspoon rosemary, dried
1   teaspoon oregano, dried
1   teaspoon salt
$\frac{1}{2}$ teaspoon cayenne pepper
$\frac{1}{2}$ cup fish stock, recipe found in the *Cooking Stock* section
3   medium yellow onions
3   medium tomatoes, sliced thin *

* *Only add for Weight Loss Program A*

Make three to four 2-inch long, $\frac{1}{2}$-inch deep, evenly spaced slits along the top of each salmon fillet. In a small bowl, whisk together mustard, lemon juice, thyme, rosemary, oregano, salt and pepper. Add salmon and turn to coat both sides. Cover with plastic wrap and refrigerate for at least 1 hour, the longer the better.

Preheat the oven to 450 degrees. Coat a shallow baking dish wit cooking spray. Add fish stock. Arrange onion on the bottom of the pan and place tomato slices on top. Place salmon on top of tomatoes and pour remaining marinade over salmon. Cover with foil and roast 7-8 minutes. Remove foil and continue roasting for 7-8 minutes, until fish is fork-tender.

Mediterranean Mahi-Mahi

1   teaspoon thyme, dried
$1/2$ teaspoon salt
$1/2$ teaspoon garlic powder
$1/2$ teaspoon ground black pepper
1   teaspoon ground sage
$1/2$ teaspoon fennel seed
$1/2$ teaspoon onion powder
1   teaspoon rosemary
$1/2$ teaspoon coriander
$1/2$ teaspoon dill weed
1   teaspoon oregano, dried
$1/2$ teaspoon ground ginger
2   bay leaves, crushed
$1/2$ teaspoon mint, dried
1   lemon, squeeze for juice
4   Mahi-Mahi fillets, 1" thick
$1/2$ cup fish stock, use recipe found in the *Cooking Stock* section
      rosemary sprigs
      whole mint leaves

Combine all ingredients in a small bowl to make a rub. Rinse fish and pat dry. Drizzle fillets with lemon juice and sprinkle rub generously. Transfer to food storage bag and set aside for at least 1 hour.

Preheat oven to 350 degrees. Place fillets in a baking dish coated with cooking spray. Add fish stock and cover with foil. Bake for 30 minutes. Transfer to serving platter and garnish with whole mint leaves and rosemary sprigs.

Steamed Lobster with Tomatoes, Saffron, Basil and Thyme

2   lobsters, $1^1/_2$ pounds each
1   cup water
1   lemon, cut into 4 wedges
2   tomatoes, chopped *
1   small bunch fresh basil
1   pinch saffron
$^1/_2$ teaspoon fresh thyme, chopped fine
    salt
    ground black pepper

* *Only add for Weight Loss Program A*

Rinse the lobsters and slide a skewer along the underside of each tail to keep the tails straight. In a large pot, bring the water and lemon wedges to a rapid boil. Place lobsters in the pot and cover tightly. Steam for 4 minutes. Remove when lobsters are bright red. Remove meat from the shells and slice each tail into 5 or 6 medallions; cover and set aside. Leave the claw meat whole.

Strain the lobster steaming liquid into a small saucepan and add the tomatoes, basil, saffron, and thyme. Simmer. Add salt and pepper to taste. Reheat the reserved lobster (if cold) and arrange in a large serving bowl. Ladle in the tomato broth and serve immediately.

Fancy Fillets

2   tablespoons green onions, chopped
2   tablespoons parsley, chopped
1   cup fish stock, use recipe found in the *Cooking Stock* section
4   boneless fillets of firm, white-fleshed fish, such as bass,
     halibut, pompano, flounder or sole, 6 ounces each, 1" thick
1   lemon, cut into 4 wedges

Coat the bottom of a large skillet with cooking spray. Sauté onions and parsley over medium heat. Add fish stock and bring to a slow simmer. Add fillets; cook 1 minute. Cover the pan with foil and finish in the oven until the fish is tender; flesh should be opaque. Remove foil and transfer fillets to serving platter. Drizzle with lemon juice and garnish with lemon wedges.

Steamed Fish

4   boneless fillets of firm, white-fleshed fish, such as halibut,
     pompano, flounder, bass, or sole, 6 ounces each, 1" thick
$^1/_4$ teaspoon salt
$^1/_4$ teaspoon ground black pepper
2   limes, sliced thin green chutney, use recipe found in the
     Chutney section
$^1/_4$ cup fish stock, use recipe found in the *Cooking Stock* section

Season fillets with salt and pepper. Place 2 slices of lime on each and spoon chutney over the top; press gently. Place a fillet in the center of each piece of foil. Before sealing the packet, pour 2 tablespoons fish stock over fillets. Fold sides of foil towards the center and fold over loose ends to seal. Fill a large pot with 1 $^1/_2$ inches of water. Place a steaming rack or bamboo steamer over it. Bring to a boil. Arrange packets in steamer and cover with lid. Steam fish until flaky and cooked through, about 15 minutes. Serve immediately.

Broiled Salmon with Lemon and Capers

2   teaspoons lemon pepper seasoning
2   teaspoons dill
2   cloves garlic, minced
4   teaspoons capers, divided
4   salmon fillets or any other boneless, firm fish, 6 ounces each,
    $1/_2$-1" thick
    salt
    ground black pepper
2   lemons, sliced into 12 thin slices
4   teaspoons fresh lemon juice, divided

Combine all dry ingredients in a small bowl. Sprinkle $1/_4$ of the mixture on each fillet. Arrange fillets on a baking sheet coated with cooking spray. Season with salt and pepper to taste and place three lemon slices on top of each. Broil on a rack set 4-5 inches from the heat for 5 minutes, or until just cooked through. Flesh should be opaque. Transfer to a serving platter or individual plates. Drizzle with lemon juice. Serve immediatly.

Salmon Packets

1   cup snow peas *
4   salmon fillets, 6 ounces each, $1/2$" thick
1   teaspoon fresh dill, chopped
1   teaspoon fresh basil, chopped
1   teaspoon fresh thyme, chopped
1   teaspoon fresh parsley, chopped
4   teaspoons fresh lemon juice
2   teaspoons ground ginger
    salt
    ground black pepper
2   large carrots, sliced thin *
1   small zucchini, sliced medium
4   tablespoons fish stock, divided, use recipe found in the *Cooking Stock* section

* *Only add for Weight Loss Program A*

Preheat oven to 350 degrees. Blanch peas in boiling water for 30 seconds and drain. Plunge peas into cold water for 30 seconds and drain; set aside. Rinse fillets and pat dry; set aside. Combine dill, thyme, parsley, and basil in a small bowl.

Tear 4 large pieces of foil (8x10) and place one fillet in the center of each. Sprinkle one teaspoon of lemon juice and $1/2$ teaspoon ginger over each fillet, and season with salt and pepper to taste. Top each fillet with $1/4$ of each vegetable and add 1 teaspoon fish stock. Fold foil from sides to the center and fold over the loose ends to seal.

Arrange foil packets on a baking sheet. Bake for 15 minutes or until salmon is just cooked through. Be careful not to overcook. To serve, place a packet on each of four plates, open and sprinkle with fresh herb mixture.

Sautéed Sardines over Wilted Baby Arugula
Weight Loss Program A Only

2   bags baby arugula greens
2   pounds fresh sardines or small smelts, cleaned
1   pinch salt
1   pinch ground black pepper
2   tablespoons fresh lemon juice
    lemon wedges

Rinse arugula, drain and set aside. Rinse sardines, drain and pat dry; set aside. Combine sardines, salt, pepper, and lemon juice in a bowl. Preheat oven to 350 degrees. With a slotted spoon, transfer to a sardines to skillet well coated with cooking spray heated over high medium heat. Sauté until golden brown.

Transfer to serving platter lined with arugula. Season with a little salt and pepper to taste and garnish with lemon wedges.

POULTRY

Indian Spiced Chicken

4   chicken breasts, boneless and skinless
1$\frac{1}{2}$ teaspoons curry powder
$\frac{1}{2}$ teaspoon garlic salt
$\frac{1}{4}$ teaspoon ground black pepper
$\frac{1}{2}$ teaspoon ground ginger
$\frac{1}{8}$ teaspoon ground turmeric
$\frac{1}{8}$ teaspoon ground cinnamon
1   tablespoon grated orange rind
1   green onion, sliced thin
2   tablespoons fresh squeezed orange juice
$\frac{1}{2}$ bag baby spinach
2   cinnamon sticks, halved
2   medium oranges, sliced

Rinse chicken and pat dry. Place chicken in a shallow baking dish coated with cooking spray and set aside. In a dry skillet, toast curry over medium-low heat for 3 minutes. Mix with garlic salt, pepper, ginger, turmeric, cinnamon, rind, onions, and juice. Pour mixture over chicken and refrigerate for 1 hour.

Preheat oven to 375 degrees. Cover with foil and bake for 20 minutes. Remove foil and bake for another 15 minutes. Transfer to serving dish lined with spinach. Garnish with orange slices and cinnamon sticks.

Spicy roasted chicken or turkey breasts

2 teaspoons chili powder
1 teaspoon ground cumin
1 teaspoon salt
1 packet sweetener
$\frac{1}{4}$ teaspoon cayenne pepper
$\frac{1}{4}$ teaspoon white pepper
4 chicken or turkey breasts, skin on
1 medium red bell pepper
1 medium green bell pepper
1 medium yellow bell pepper
1 pound whole green beans, fresh with ends snapped off *
$\frac{1}{3}$ cup water

Only add for Weight Loss Program A

Combine all dry ingredients is a small bowl. Rub evenly over the breasts. Cover and refrigerate up to 24 hours.

Preheat oven to 325 degrees. Coat the bottom of a large baking dish with cooking spray. Place breast into baking dish skin side up. Clean and remove seeds from bell peppers. Cut into strips and add to baking dish with green beans. Pour water to bottom of dish and cover with foil. Bake for 20 minutes, then remove foil. Remove peppers, cover, and set aside until ready to serve. Continue to cook breasts until light, golden brown.

Rosemary Chicken/Turkey

4	chicken or turkey breasts, skin on
2	teaspoons fresh rosemary
	or
1	teaspoon rosemary, dried
$^1/_4$	teaspoon salt
$^1/_4$	teaspoon ground black pepper
4	stalks celery
6	small yellow onions
2	cups baby carrots, fresh or frozen *
$^1/_2$	cup fresh squeezed orange juice

* Only add for Weight Loss Program A

Preheat oven to 375 degrees. Coat a roasting pan with cooking spray and place chicken in it, skin side up. Sprinkle with rosemary, salt, and pepper. Cut celery into chunks. Peel onions and cut in half. Add vegetables to chicken, pour orange juice over all, and cover with foil. Bake for 30 minutes, then remove foil and bake until chicken is light, golden brown.

Chicken Piccata

2 pounds chicken breast cutlets
$1/2$ teaspoon marjoram, crumbled fine
$1/4$ teaspoon salt
1 teaspoon flour
$1/2$ lemon, peeled and juiced
$1/2$ clove garlic, minced
1 tablespoon parsley, chopped
   lemon slices

Lightly dust cutlets with flour and sprinkle both sides with marjoram and salt. Spray a medium skillet with cooking spray. Place cutlets in skillet and sprinkle with lemon peel, garlic, and parsley. Sauté in hot skillet 2 to 3 minutes on each side. Transfer to serving platter. Sprinkle cutlets with lemon juice. Garnish with lemon slices.

Simple Chicken or Turkey Breasts

4 boneless chicken breasts, skin on
   or
2 turkey breasts, skin on
   Adobo Seasoning (green top found in the international foods
      aisle)
1 tablespoon ground sage
1 pinch ground black pepper
$1/3$ cup water
   fresh sage sprigs

Preheat oven to 350 degrees. Coat a baking dish with cooking spray. Rinse breasts and pat dry. Shake on the Adobo seasoning generously. Follow with sage and pepper. Add water to the bottom of the dish and cover with foil. Bake for 20 minutes, then remove foil and bake another 15 minutes or until breasts are golden brown. Transfer to a serving platter and garnish with sage sprigs.

Citrus-Herb Chicken or Turkey

5   tablespoons fresh squeezed orange juice
2   tablespoons lime juice
2   heaping tablespoons oregano
1   teaspoon ground cumin
1   teaspoon chili powder
1   clove garlic, chopped
1   large orange, peeled and sectioned
    salt
    ground black pepper
4   boneless chicken breasts, skin on
    or
2   turkey breasts, skin on

In a food processor or blender, combine all ingredients except the chicken, add salt and pepper to taste, and puree until smooth. Pre-heat the oven to 350 degrees. Coat the bottom of a large baking dish with cooking spray. Arrange chicken in the dish and brush with half the citrus-herb mixture. Cover with foil. Bake the chicken, turning once and brushing occasionally with the remaining mixture for 30 minutes. Transfer to serving patter and season with salt and pepper to taste. Garnish with oranges.

VEAL

Veal with Pepper-Pear Relish*
Weight Loss Program A Only

4	veal loin or rib chops, cut into 1" slices
$3/_4$	teaspoon salt, divided
$1/_4$	teaspoon coarse black pepper
1	large red bell pepper, cut into $1/_2$" pieces
1	large green bell pepper, cut into $1/_2$" pieces
$1/_2$	cup yellow onion, chopped
2	tablespoons jalapeno pepper, minced
1	tablespoon fresh ginger, minced
2	medium pears, peeled and cut into $1/_2$ pieces
6	tablespoons fresh lemon juice, divided
1	cup water
1	packet sweetener
1	teaspoon grated lemon peel
1	tablespoon cornstarch
2	tablespoons cilantro, chopped
	cilantro sprigs
	lemon twists

Place veal on broiler rack coated with cooking spray so surface of meat is 4 inches away from heat. Broil 15 minutes for medium, turning once. Season with salt and pepper. Heat cooking sprayed skillet over medium heat. Add bell peppers, onion, jalapeno pepper and ginger. Cook 10 minutes stirring occasionally. Do not cover. Stir in pears, 4 tablespoons lemon juice, water, sweetener, lemon peel and remaining $1/_2$ teaspoon salt. Simmer 5 minutes or until pears are tender, stirring occasionally. Mix cornstarch and water to thicken, if desired. Remove from heat and stir in remaining 2 tablespoons lemon juice and chopped cilantro. Arrange veal on serving platter and spoon pear relish on top. Garnish with cilantro sprigs and lemon twists.

Veal Piccata *
Weight Loss Program A Only

1   pound veal cutlets
1   tablespoon cornstarch
$^1/_2$ teaspoon salt
$^1/_2$ teaspoon garlic salt
$^1/_4$ teaspoon paprika
2   tablespoons capers, drained
2   tablespoons fresh lemon juice
     ground black pepper
1   medium lemon, sliced
1   teaspoon parsley, dried

Dredge veal in cornstarch, salt, garlic salt, pepper and paprika. Spray a large skillet with cooking spray. Brown veal on both sides over medium heat. Remove to serving platter. Add capers to skillet. Stir and pour drippings over veal. Sprinkle with lemon juice. Add black pepper to taste. Garnish with lemon slices sprinkled with parsley.

Lemon Veal with Peppercorns*
Weight Loss Program A Only

1   large lemon
3   cloves garlic, crushed
2   teaspoons peppercorns
$\frac{1}{2}$ teaspoon salt
2   veal chops, 7 ounces each, trimmed of all fat

Juice the lemon and set aside. Combine garlic, peppercorn, salt and half of lemon juice in a shallow dish. Add veal chops, turning to coat both sides. Press some peppercorns into each chop. Refrigerate 1 hour, then let stand at room temperature for 30 minutes.

Heat a skillet coated with cooking spray over medium heat. Add veal chops and sear on both sides until browned. Discard all but 1 teaspoon drippings from pan. Reduce heat to low, cover and cook another 10 minutes, or until tender. Transfer to a serving platter. Add remaining lemon juice to the pan and simmer. Spoon over chops and serve. Garnish with more peppercorns.

Sautéed Veal Scallops*
Weight Loss Program A Only

2   tablespoons flour
1   teaspoon garlic powder
$^1/_2$ teaspoon salt
$^1/_2$ teaspoon ground black pepper
1   pound veal scallops, $^1/_4$" thick, pounded flat
1   heaping tablespoon fresh basil, chopped
2   tablespoons fresh lemon juice

Combine flour, garlic powder, salt, and pepper in a shallow dish. Drizzle scallops with lemon juice and dust each with flour mixture. Shake off excess. Coat a large skillet with cooking spray and heat over medium heat. Sauté the scallops turning frequently until tender. Transfer to serving platter. Garnish with fresh basil.

SNACKS

Turkey Roll Ups

2-3 turkey breast slices, fresh or deli lettuce
    toothpicks
    fat-free salad dressing (ranch works well)
    mustard

On a single slice of turkey breast, place a slice of lettuce that fits the size of the turkey breast. Roll the turkey breast around the lettuce and use a toothpick to secure it. Before eating, optionally dip the roll into the fat-free salad dressing or mustard.

Tangy Cucumbers

1   cucumber
    salt
    ground black pepper
    vinegar

Peel and slice a cucumber into $1/4$" circular sections. Place the sections in a container. Sprinkle with salt and pepper to taste. Generously pour vinegar over the sections.

Baked Apple

1 medium apple (Macintosh, Fuji, Red Delicious or Gala)
   cinnamon
2 packets sweetener

Peel the apple and slice it in circular sections. Place the sections in a microwavable container. Sprinkle with cinnamon and sweetener to taste. Microwave for 1 minute or until soft.

Sweet Strawberries

6 strawberries
2 packets sweetener

Slice strawberries into thin sections and place them in a storage container. Sprinkle with sweetener to taste. Cover and refrigerate strawberries for at least 1 hour.

Warmed Grapefruit

1 grapefruit
3 strawberries

Cut the grapefruit in half. On a cutting board, slice the strawberries and mash with the back side of a spoon. Place the strawberries on top of the grapefruit. Microwave for 1 minute or until warm.

Appendix C

FOOD DIARY

K eeping a *Food Diary* of all the food and drink you consume each day can be very helpful. This diary should be kept with you at all times. Write down all food or drinks before you eat or drink them. Once you write something down, if you think that you should not consume it, leave it out and mark through the entry.

A blank sample *Food Diary* is on the next page.

Food Diary

Date: _____ Day of the week: _____

	Breakfast	Lunch	Dinner	Snacks
Meats				
Vegetables				
Fruits				
Other				

I drank this much water today: _____

Recipe Index

Sole 185
Spinach 166, 172, 189
Squash 176
Stock, chicken 157
Stock, fish 158, 182, 183, 185, 187
Stock, vegetable 156, 171, 173, 177
Strawberries 150, 167, 199
Sweetener 149

T
Tangerines 152, 166
Tarragon 156, 157, 158, 175
Thyme 151, 156, 157, 158, 177, 179, 182, 183, 184, 187
Tomatoes 155, 161, 162, 163, 165, 169, 173, 182, 184
Tuna 162, 165, 180
Turkey 152, 164, 168, 190, 191, 192, 193, 198
Turkey breast slices 198
Turmeric 189

V
Veal 194, 195, 196, 197
Vinaigrette 150
Vinegar
    150, 152, 159, 160, 166, 169, 170, 175, 176, 177, 180,
    198

W
Wasabi paste 180

Z
Zucchini 174, 187

GENERAL INDEX

A
Aerobics xxx, 49, 86, 93, 98, 99, 104, 105, 126
Alcohol 76, 81, 114
American Society of Bariatric Physicians
     xiv, xv, xxii, xxiii, 69, 89, 95, 101, 108, 127, 130, 134
Anemia 80, 131
Anniversary 123
Anorexic 126
Appetite suppressants
     69, 88, 94, 100, 107, 128, 129, 134 (see also "Diet pills")
Apple 85, 92, 98, 104, 106, 113, 115, 119, 141
Arthritis xxiv, 44, 46, 48, 133, 145
Asparagus 85, 92, 98, 104

B
Bariatric surgery 131
Beale, Lisa M. xv, 143
Beale, Robert S., Jr., M.D. xiv, xv, 88, 94, 100, 107, 129, 143
Beans 59, 60, 61, 75, 85, 137
Beets 85
Bicycle xxx, 49, 86, 93, 99, 105, 126
Bingeing 83, 87, 90, 94, 96, 100, 102, 106, 146

Weight, goal
    35, 36, 37, 42, 47, 51, 105, 107, 110, 139, 140, 141
Weight, healthy
    xxi, xxviii-xxx, 36, 37, 38, 39, 42, 43, 45, 46, 47, 48,
    49, 50, 51, 52, 67, 71, 83, 90, 96, 102, 107, 122, 125,
    136, 143, 145, 146
Weight Loss Program
    xxii, 35, 46, 48, 49, 52, 56, 57, 62, 67, 68, 69, 70,
    71, 72, 73, 75, 76, 77, 78, 83, 84, 86, 87, 88, 90, 91,
    92, 93, 94, 96, 97, 98, 99, 100, 102, 103, 104, 105,
    106, 107, 109, 110, 111, 112, 113, 114, 116, 117, 118,
    119, 122, 123, 124, 127, 128, 130, 132, 135, 136, 139,
    140, 141, 142, 143
Weight Loss Strategies 35, 45, 46, 109
Weight, obese xxvii, 37, 40, 42, 45-48
Weight, seriously obese xxvii, 37, 41, 42, 45-48
Weight, unhealthy xxvii, 124
Weights, lifting 49, 86, 93, 99, 105, 126
Will power 46

Y
Yogurt xxvii, 47, 75, 137

Z
Zucchini 85

Book Order Form

Fax orders: 202-478-0686. Send a copy of this form.

Phone orders: Call 866-211-DIET toll free. Have your credit card ready.

E-mail orders: orders@TheDietSolutions.com

Postal orders: Make your check or money order payable to *The Diet Solutions, L.L.P.* and send to:

> The Diet Solutions, L.L.P.
> P.O. Box 65306
> Washington, D.C. 20035-5306

Orders over 50 books: Call 866-211-DIET

YES, I want _____ copies of *The Black Diet Doctor's Solution For Black Women* for $24.95 each.

Include $4.00 shipping and handling for one book, and $2.00 for each additional book. Washington, D.C. residents must include applicable sales tax.

Payment in U.S. funds must accompany order.
Name: _____
Address: _____
City/State/Zip Code: _____
Phone: _____
E-mail: _____

My check or money order for $_____ is enclosed.
Please charge my ___ Visa ___ Mastercard ___Discover
Card number: _____
Name on card: _____ Exp. date: _____
Signature: _____